COWBOYS AND INDIAN
– BOOK 3 –
SPECIALIST IN THE FIELD

SANDIP V. MATHUR, M.D.

Genre: Creative Non-Fiction

ISBN: 979-8-9873351-0-9

Designed by Tinyah M. Hawkins/Goofidity Designs

Cover Photograph by Michelle Hanna

Printed in the USA

Published by TexasStarTrading.com
174 Cypress Street
Abilene, Texas 79601
info@texasstartrading.com
(325) 672-9696

To my wife and family
In memory of my sister

TABLE OF CONTENTS

PREFACE

I completed my formal training in internal medicine and gastroenterology in Houston in 1995. I was keen to start my medical practice but I was on a student visa. The Hotspur medical center in central Texas was unable to recruit local doctors. The hospital board interviewed me and offered us green cards if I worked in Hotspur for three years.

The hospital had been struggling financially but the other doctors and I were able to turn things around. Although I am a specialist, I worked as a general practitioner for two years and built up my practice. In my third year, the hospital leased specialty equipment for me and I started doing procedures like upper endoscopies and colonoscopies in the operating rooms of the hospital.

In endoscopic procedures, thin flexible fiber-optic tubes are used to examine the stomach and colon. In upper endoscopy, the patient is sedated and the endoscope is passed through the mouth and into the food pipe, the stomach, and the first part of the small intestine, also called the duodenum. A camera at the tip allows the inner lining to be seen on a TV monitor. Channels in the endoscope allow us to pass other instruments through the endoscope and take biopsies of suspicious areas and treat bleeding ulcers and leaking blood vessels. Colonoscopy is similar; it is the examination of the large intestine or colon with a longer endoscope. It is used for the same reasons but there is also the great advantage of being able to remove pre-cancerous growths called polyps.

This book is an account of my third year in rural Texas. I continued to practice general medicine but spent more time in my specialty. There were many exciting challenges and some setbacks, but I persevered. In my other books, I have written about my first two years. This book continues the narrative into the third year, when I strove to be a gastroenterologist rather than an internist.

The political correctness of cities is absent in small towns; the American psyche lies bare. We learned much about our new country by living in Hotspur. The townspeople were initially wary but soon became warm and welcoming. We accepted the scrutiny and honesty of our neighbors, many of whom remain close to this day. My wife and our two daughters embraced Hotspur, as did I. We came to love the town and the people dearly. They took us into their hearts and homes.

These events happened over twenty-five years ago. These accounts, like the two preceding books, are based on memory. I have deliberately changed names and details, including those of my family, to maintain privacy. Although based on true occurrences, events and individuals have been altered and reconfigured, so this is not an accurate or precise retelling.

As I look back on those formative years, I am grateful for the many wonderful opportunities that came my way, and my good fortune to have been in Texas when they arrived. I also realize my mistakes and shortcomings and am humbled that my patients, family, and colleagues were so kind and understanding. I could have done a lot of things better, but I couldn't have chosen a better place to live and practice.

Through my writing, I hope to convey the friendship, love, and respect that emerged on both sides. I hope to share the challenges, thrills and rewards of my third year in Texas.

Sandip V. Mathur

CHAPTER 1

DANGER DEAD AHEAD

I knew it was cancer the minute I saw it.

It was a huge polyp, like a giant black mushroom, and it blocked the way forward. The surface was irregular and coated with thick green mucus. I washed it with water and suctioned off the debris. The mucus coat quickly dissolved, revealing a raw crimson lining with twisted blood vessels. I washed it again, slowly, so as to avoid damaging the blood vessels.

I was alarmed. I studied the polyp after cleaning it.

The top of the polyp was definitely malignant, but the stalk was smooth. It was possible that the cancer had not invaded the stalk. All I had to do was to cut the base of the stalk; I could remove the cancer before it had a chance to infiltrate down the stalk and spread. Cutting the base of the stalk could solve the problem and save my patient an operation.

The malignant mass had to be removed, and I had done many similar cases before. But those cases had been in Houston and London. Now I was in a remote part of Texas with no backup. Could I do it safely? A large growth like this could have robust arteries in the stalk that might bleed ferociously. What if I cut the polyp and couldn't stop the bleeding?

We were in an operating room in Hotspur, Texas, performing a colonoscopy. Our patient, Emily Trueblood, was sedated and lying on her left side, and the endoscope was in her colon, her large intestine. The interior of the colon was displayed on a grainy screen. The nurse, Penny Merriwether, and I gawked at it. The growth wobbled with the irrigation. I stopped flushing, suctioned the water out, and pumped in carbon dioxide gas to stretch the colon open. I inched closer to the growth and suctioned again. My mind raced.

Dare I cut this massive polyp?

The suctioning suddenly wrenched the polyp against the tip of the endoscope and everything went red. I washed again and re-inflated. The polyp fell back and rotated. I saw the other side of the head. It was irregular, with two smaller lobes. The gas I had just pumped in moved out abruptly and the lining of the colon collapsed around the polyp like a shroud. I pumped in more gas, but the patient expelled it out again. I kept pushing in more gas but the colonic lining remained collapsed. I called out in frustration.

"I can't do anything if I can't keep it inflated!" I cried.

Penny was agitated. She shook her head and waved her hands in frustration.

"I don't know what to do! What're you going to do, Doc?" Penny asked. "And, anyway, how're we going to keep it open?"

I calmed myself and remembered what I had done in the past.

"She's lying on her side, I bet that's compressing her sigmoid colon. Let's roll her onto her back," I decided.

Penny jumped into action. We straightened our patients' legs and rolled her onto her back. I inflated again. Penny rubbed Emily's ankles soothingly.

"Bless her heart, that polyp looks like vile corruption on top of vile corruption," she declared.

I racked my brain furiously.

In Houston or London, I would have had no hesitation removing that polyp. Had it bled, I would have injected adrenaline or clamped it with a metal clip. And I could have called a surgeon to bail me out, if necessary. But we were in Hotspur, sixty miles from the closest ICU!

I took a deep breath.

"It looks really bad," Penny said.

I nodded.

I could withdraw the scope and send her to a gastroenterologist in Abilene, that might be the safest option. But that would mean I had not examined the rest of the colon, and I had left my patient with a cancer that was poised to spread.

There was something else.

And it would appear that I was unsure of my abilities. Word might get around that I wasn't able to handle anything complicated.

That bothered me.

"Let's get the heck out of here before we get our asses whupped," Penny declared, with a shudder. "It just looks meaner than evil. Bad deal!"

But if I didn't do what I was trained to do, I would lose credibility.

I took a deep breath.

"It looks bad," I agreed, "But it does have a smooth stalk that looks uninvolved. Give me a snare, Penny. I'm going to cut that stalk!"

Penny was aghast.

"What? Doctor, are you *serious*? Are you going to mess with that monster?" she asked, alarmed.

I didn't know what to say. I reconsidered my options quickly.

Was I jeopardizing my patient out of vanity? I could just take a biopsy and abandon the procedure. Or I could remove the polyp and complete my examination, like a real specialist.

I put my hand out.

"Snare, please," I said.

Penny jumped back and shook her head vigorously.

"Oh, no! No, no! You're really going to cut it, aren't you? Don't do it!" she pleaded.

I bristled. I never like being told what to do, even if it's undeniably sensible. Most doctors, I like to think, have brittle egos and hate being held back. We keep pushing the limits and often take chances when we're not sure of success or failure. We call this *experience*. So I gazed at the screen and ignored Penny. I thought again, not as a regular physician, but as a *specialist*.

"Doctor, please just pull out now! Don't risk it!" Penny pleaded.

What I heard was, *you can't do it.*

That stung.

True, I could just take a biopsy and pull out and send her to a bigger hospital. That would be the safest thing to do. But it would prolong the process by days or weeks. Or I could use my skills and cut it out and resolve the whole matter right there.

I maneuvered the instrument. Penny hopped around in agitation.

"What are you going to do?" she asked. "I'm terrified!"

"Calm down. I'm just taking a better look at it," I said.

"Doctor, I know you're used to working in big hospitals in Houston and London. But this is little Hotspur, Texas," she pleaded.

"I know."

"We're a *tiny* yee-haw hospital in the middle of *nowhere*, Doc!"

"I realize that, Penny."

"Doc, what if you cut it off and she bleeds? You know we ain't set up for someone bleeding! We got no blood bank in our itty bitty hospital."

"We have two units of O negative blood," I grunted.

"That's *all* the blood we have in the whole county! You got to be real careful. Don't bite off more'n you can chew!"

I moved the tip of the scope from side to side at the base of the polyp.

"If she bleeds like crazy she could have a heart attack," Penny went on.

"I realize that."

"Or a stroke. She could have a stroke."

"Very unlikely."

Penny crossed her arms and glared at me.

"I'm sorry, I don't fancy doing CPR here or in the ambulance to Baptist Hospital. She could bleed out!"

"You think I don't know that?"

"She could *die*. People have *died* from medical mistakes. Why are you pushing the scope around?"

"I'm checking to see if the stalk is smooth all around. That would mean that the cancer on the top has not invaded the stalk," I explained.

"The stock?"

"No, I mean the stalk, the smooth tube which connects the cancer to the lining of the colon."

"Oh, a *stalk?* You mean, like the stalk of a flower?" Penny asked, and stepped closer to the screen.

"The *stalk*. This polyp has a decent *stalk*. So we can cut it," I said, with clenched teeth.

"Sometimes, I don't even understand what you say, your accent. I'm just an average surgical nurse, and that looks like a big, fat cancer. So I say, just leave it alone. Ship her to Abilene or Dallas, Doc," Penny pleaded.

I adopted what I thought was a reassuring tone.

"Don't worry, I realize this is our first week of doing colonoscopies in Hotspur. I'm going to guide you through it," I said.

"You're taking a mighty big chance," she muttered. "I guess it's good that you got confidence."

"I do have experience," I admitted.

"Bet you were top of your class!" Penny said.

I remembered my program director. "Mathur's not the best, but he's not the worst either. If it was my family, I would pick someone else over Mathur," he had said.

I decided to change the subject quickly. I pointed to a packet on the table.

"That's the snare forceps. Open it and hand it to me."

Penny did so reluctantly.

"I'm just checking it, getting a better assessment," I said, soothingly.

"Okay, then," Penny smiled.

"Good. Now I feed the tip of the snare into the scope at this end and you'll see the tip come out the other end. Watch the screen."

The tip of the snare emerged promptly.

"So the snare is inside her now?" Penny asked.

"Yes. The *tip* of the snare forceps is inside her, in her sigmoid colon. The sigmoid colon is in the lower left side of the abdomen."

"I *know* that, Doctor."

I poked the head of the polyp with the tip of the snare. It buckled and bled a little.

"Ow! Ow! Don't do that! You made it bleed!" Penny recoiled.

I prodded the top of the polyp. It toppled backwards and slipped away, revealing the thick white cord.

"Is that thick white tube the stalk?" Penny asked.

"Yes."

"Looks pretty thick, about a quarter inch, you reckon?"

"Yes."

"Is that good or bad, that it's got a stalk?"

"It's good. *Very* good. It looks like there's a pretty good stalk. Maybe we can cut it off with our snare," I said.

Penny was horrified.

"Whoa! No, no! You said you were just checking it!"

"I know. I was checking it out to see if it had a stalk, to see if I could safely cut it."

Penny shook her head emphatically.

"Cut it? Cut that huge, nasty thing? Are you crazy?" she shrieked.

"It's got a decent stalk. I can cut it off."

"But what if there's an artery inside that stalk?"

"Inject it with adrenaline."

"Will that work?"

"Yes, it does."

"What if it doesn't?"

"I've done this procedure hundreds of times, Penny. I can handle it."

"Doctor, we haven't done this sort of procedure here in Hotspur. Maybe you did those things all the time in Houston and London but this is Hotspur! I refuse!"

I was angry, but I held back.

"I understand your reluctance," I said. "But I'm a specialist. I've done these procedures many, many times. I know how to deal with it."

Penny was still unconvinced. She held up her hands and shook her head vigorously. She took a step back.

"We've got no ICU, no surgeon, no fancy equipment, no nothing!" she said.

I hesitated. I looked at the screen again.

"No back-up, no anesthesia, no CT!"

"I realize that."

"We're out in the sticks with nothing, but *nothing* to help us! I'm scared!"

Penny was bubbling with agitation. She took another step back. I panicked. I needed her help.

"I know, I know. But I really think I could cut that polyp out. I've done it so many times, on even bigger polyps."

"No! Don't do it, Doctor! Don't do it!" Penny urged me. She did not return to my side.

A familiar voice growled behind me. I jumped.

"She's right, Einstein. Don't do it," it advised. I turned around and peered into the darkness.

"Karl! What are you doing here?" I said.

"Question is, what are *you* doing here?" Karl countered.

"Obviously I'm doing a colonoscopy. She's got this big polyp and I think it's malignant."

"Swell. So you made the diagnosis. Now get the H E double hockey-sticks out of there and pack her off to Abilene!" Karl thundered.

"I can remove that polyp!" I protested. "I've done lots of polyps like this one."

"Sure you have, O Grand Piano, but this is not your fancy-ass Royal Hospital of London or the Houston medical city, savvy? You cut that polyp, she bleeds like a stuck pig, then we got only two units of O negative to get her to Abilene with."

"She won't bleed much, I'm pretty sure."

"You realize she's also a Board member?" he added.

"Yes."

"One of your biggest supporters?"

"Yes."

"So why are you taking a chance? Why are you trying to be a hero?"

"I'm a specialist. I can do this," I repeated.

"You mess with her, you'll get sued, Einstein."

I was silent.

"Didn't think of that, did you? She's royalty around here. She's going to sue the pants off you, I'll bet the judge'll be her uncle and the jurors all go to her church and you'll be out on your ass."

I exhaled. Karl was right.

"Give up, man. You're taking a shitload of risk and what does it get you? Nothing!"

Karl shook my shoulder.

"Don't be an idiot. Get your ass out of there," he advised.

My mouth parched and my heart raced. I didn't know what to say. Karl sensed my hesitation.

"The rest of the Hospital Board will nail you to the wall if you screw up!" Karl added, his voice strangely cheerful.

I gritted my teeth and glared at him. Karl laughed.

"You are a real piece of work!" he declared.

"I *can* remove that polyp. I've done it before many times, really, and some even bigger."

Karl shook his head.

"Negative. First rule of medicine is, cover your ass," he said.

"It's got a decent stalk," I reasoned.

Karl sighed and shook his head.

"Yeah. Decent stalk with a decent artery that's gonna bleed like stink."

"I can stop the bleeding, if it happens."

Karl shook his head.

"Listen, moron. No one would like to see you fail more than me. And I'm telling you, just forget it," he advised.

His advice had the opposite effect on me. I *had* to prove myself.

"I *can* do it," I repeated, grimly.

Karl stared at me in astonishment. He shrugged.

"It's your funeral, man. Don't say I didn't tell you," he said.

* * *

I washed the polyp again and photographed it. I weighed my options. I wished Karl would leave. I looked back at Penny.

"Lost your nerve?" Karl inquired, pleasantly.

"No," I replied.

"Sounds like you're scared."

I cleared my throat.

"No, I'm not. I can do this. I'm trained in this and I have the experience."

"Yeah, that's going to really impress the jury," Karl said. "You complete moron."

"Doctor, don't let Dr. Karl push you!" Penny blurted.

"Who asked you, Nurse Ratchett?" Karl snapped.

"Open the snare, Penny," I ordered.

"But I agree with Dr. Becker!" Penny added, hastily. "Don't do it!"

"I *can* do this. Open the snare!" I said.

"I'm warning you, Doctor!" Penny repeated.

She operated the snare reluctantly. A large metal lasso appeared. I tried to wriggle it over the top of the polyp, but it kept slipping off.

"Your hands are shaking, brother!" Karl pointed out.

I twisted the endoscope from side to side and jiggled the snare over the top of the polyp.

"Penny, connect the snare to cautery," I ordered.

"We got some problems with our cautery, Doctor," Penny mumbled.

"*What?* Why didn't you tell me earlier?"

"I didn't expect you would actually want to *do* anything. Figured you were just going to look and then come out."

"I want to snare this big polyp and I want to cauterize it so it doesn't bleed. And you're telling me the cautery doesn't work?"

"Let me check the dang cautery," Karl snorted.

He fiddled with the buttons and turned the power off and on.

"This cautery unit is a piece of junk," he declared.

He disconnected the wall plug, then re-connected it.

"Try it again," he said.

Penny inserted the snare electrode into several slots, one after another. She checked the monitor anxiously. It remained silent.

"The monitor has *not come on*, Penny," I snapped.

"I am trying, Doctor, I'm a-trying!" she said, flustered.

"This is going to be a complete disaster," Karl smirked. He pulled up a stool and sat down. "A real dumpster fire!"

"Switch it off and try again!" I ordered.

Penny complied. We waited a minute then tried all the possible connections again.

"It's still not working, Penny!" I shouted.

"I can't help it, Doctor! I don't know what to do."

"How am I supposed to remove a polyp if there's no cautery?"

"I'm sorry, Doctor. I just don't know what else to do," she wailed.

Karl snorted.

"Give up, Einstein. This just isn't your day."

I gazed at the screen. The polyp bobbed back and forth victoriously, glazing over with blood and mucus.

"Get me adrenaline, ten cc of one in ten thousand adrenaline!" I ordered.

Penny opened her mouth but said nothing.

"We don't even have adrenaline?" I asked, astonished, "We don't have cautery, and we don't even have adrenaline?"

"Told you. You're up shit creek without a paddle. Literally," Karl snorted.

"We don't have adrenaline here in the room. But it's in the pharmacy. Be right back," Penny said, and shot out of the room.

"What good's that going to do when you don't have cautery?" asked Karl.

"One alternative to cauterization is to cut the base without cauterization, and inject the area with adrenaline before and after cutting it."

"So you're going to just slice it off without burning the stump?"

"Yes."

"*Seriously?*"

"Yes. I plan to put a clip as well, to pinch the tissues together afterwards, like a staple."

Karl exhaled loudly.

"Listen, Einstein. Like I said, no one would be happier than me to see you get your royal ass kicked out of here, no one, okay? But even I can't let you do this. Give it up! You made the diagnosis. Cover yourself in glory! But now, go home. Ship her off to Abilene, and be done with it!"

I started sweating. My mouth dried up so much I could barely talk.

Karl stood up.

"Listen up, Einstein. Specialists belong in big cities, not in little po-dunk towns like Hotspur," he said.

I swallowed and licked my lips.

"I'm going to try," I croaked.

"Why?"

"Because I'm a specialist. I've got the training. I think we should do as much as we can do safely right here. Good for the patients and good for the hospital," I said. "Makes us look credible."

Karl snorted.

"Screw credibility. If something happens to her, its going to be really bad for you!" he warned. "Remember, she's on the Board. Imagine the headlines, *Hospital Board Member Killed By Overzealous Doctor!*"

He had a point. I remained silent.

"I know you, oh great Member of the Royal College of Physicians of London. Usually, you're so cautious! This isn't you! Why are you trying to be a hero? Give up already! This is way beyond you, okay?"

I was glad it was dark so Karl couldn't see me tremble. He stood up and hissed in my ear.

"Your funeral, man! Your damn *funeral!*"

Penny returned with the adrenaline drawn up in a ten cc syringe.

"Got it!" she said, waving it triumphantly.

Karl ambled to the door.

"I just came here to tell you that your pal, Dell Clawsom, is in the clinic. He's my patient, but wants to see you for some reason. So whenever you get done with this catastrophe, after you sign her death certificate and nail up her coffin, come on over to the clinic."

Karl slammed the door and left.

I changed my mind. I decided that Karl was right, and I had no stomach for a lawsuit. I decided to give up and waved to Penny to admit defeat. But Penny was transformed.

"*Yes!* Let's do this!" Penny enthused. She slammed the adrenaline into my palm.

"What? I thought you were dead against it!" I exclaimed.

Penny grabbed my wrist forcefully.

"I believe in you, Doctor. You've got all that fancy training in London and Houston, and I believe you when you say you can do this."

I was taken aback.

"You're a specialist!" Penny whooped.

I didn't know what to say.

"I believe you. You can do this without hurting sweet Emily."

I coughed nervously.

"You know how to do this without her bleeding to death," Penny said, brightly.

"Thanks," I mumbled, my voice an octave lower.

"Go on, then!" Penny urged.

I peered at her, confused.

"What happened to you?" I asked, as I removed the snare from the endoscope and replaced it with the injection catheter.

"I'm tired of seeing Dr. Karl push you around, Doctor."

"He means well," I said, defensively.

"Nah. You're this little brown dude and he's this good old white boy who's way bigger than you, just busting your chops all the time," Penny declared. "But you're finally standing up for yourself, like a real Texan, so I'm behind you all the way!"

I had always seen our conflict as a clash of titans. Apparently, it did not look like that to everyone.

"Oh," I said, crestfallen.

"You're a true blue ballsy Texan now," Penny declared.

"Oh," I repeated, further deflated.

"I'm ready to inject the adrenaline!" Penny chirped, waving the syringe.

The tip of the injection catheter emerged on the screen. My medical career balanced on it. I took a deep breath.

"Needle out!" I ordered.

Penny pushed the steel needle out of the plastic sheath. I guided the tip of the needle to the base of the stalk and jabbed it in.

"Inject two cc."

Penny injected. Adrenaline squirted from the base.

"Slowly! Slowly!"

"Yes, Doctor."

I repositioned.

"Again! One cc first, then another, but very slowly!"

My voice was becoming high-pitched.

"Yes, Doctor. Sorry for injecting too fast."

We injected again.

"Watch the polyp. It should turn pale as we constrict the blood supply."

The polyp looked exactly the same. We waited another minute. And another.

"The polyp seems to be shrinking a little, Doc."

"I'm going to complete the rest of the exam and then come back to it."

I maneuvered the endoscope past the growth and slowly advanced it all the way to the other end of the colon. No more masses. I sighed with relief.

"Now you're going to pull back, Doctor?" Penny asked.

"Yes. Very slowly. We often see polyps on the way out."

But there were no others. And when we returned to the sigmoid colon, the polyp had shrunk further.

"Well done, Doctor!" Penny said, "That looks much smaller!"

"Yes," I agreed. "Adrenaline tightens the blood vessels. The polyp looks pale and shrunken. Now I can slip the snare over it."

I passed the snare forceps through the instrument and watched the tip emerge on the screen.

"Open the snare all the way."

Penny obeyed.

I looped the snare over the top of the growth like a garland and slid it down to the bottom of the stalk.

"Okay, close the snare. But do it slowly, very slowly!"

Penny closed the snare. The loop tightened around the bottom of the stalk and the polyp shuddered.

"Good position! Close it! Close!" I barked.

"It won't close, Doctor!" Penny reported.

"Give it a little force."

"I'm closing as hard as I can!"

The polyp started swelling and turned maroon.

"Okay, open the snare!"

"Open it?" Penny was surprised.

"Yes. I'm going to change my angle."

I repositioned the snare, moving a fraction higher.

"Now close again!"

Penny struggled.

"It still won't close completely, Doctor."

"Penny, try harder."

"I am trying, Doctor!"

"I'm going to jiggle the tip to help you," I said.

"It's not helping. It's not working!" Penny wailed.

The polyp swelled up to its original dimensions but remained purple.

"It's big again, Doctor!"

"I can see that, Penny," I grimaced.

"I can't get it any tighter, Doctor."

"Try to connect to cautery again, then. Power setting should be fifteen watts, not twenty."

Penny let go of the snare. The loop opened up and slid right off the growth. I groaned. She threw her arms up.

"Sorry, but I can't do two things at once, Doctor."

Penny fumbled with the cautery machine.

"I can't see anything. I'm going to turn the lights back on."

Penny turned the lights on and tried all the connections again.

"It's still not working, Doctor," she sighed.

I was at a loss. I realized that I was failing badly. I was not able to sever the polyp stalk and if I pulled too hard, it could cause the tissue to rip off and create a giant wound. Pulling and cutting would produce more trauma and more bleeding.

* * *

Karl kicked the door open and strode in.

"Just spoke to Emily's daughter, Gwen. Guess what she said? She said her mother is an easy bleeder. Bleeds from the smallest cut."

Karl chuckled. I exhaled and mentally rehearsed my surrender speech.

"Ain't you the lucky one!"

"Bleeds like a dang pig," he added, slapping me on the shoulder.

He looked at the screen.

"It won't cut?" he guessed correctly.

"No," I admitted.

"This is great, Einstein. You got a VIP patient, you got a mother of a polyp, you got no cautery, your snare won't cut it and if you do manage to rip the darn thing off, she's an easy bleeder. I love it," Karl enthused. "You're a dead man."

"Open the snare fully!" I ordered.

I tried to slide the snare over the polyp, but it kept snagging on the back. I twisted the scope and changed the angle of the snare, but it didn't help.

"Are you going to get the snare on it sometime today?" Karl asked.

I said nothing. I stopped moving the snare. I had given up.

"Giving up?" Karl grinned.

"He's not giving up! He's going to try again," Penny said, enthusiastically. "Just you see, Dr. Becker."

She switched off the lights and grasped the snare forceps. I tried one last time. It slid over the head of the polyp and stopped at a perfect site just a little below the head, at the top of the stalk. Karl was astonished.

"What the heck?" he gagged.

"Yo! Let's do this!" Penny cried out.

I opened my mouth to tell her to stop. Karl moved in closer.

"All right, Royal Physician to the Queen of England! Show me your stuff!"

I closed my mouth. I tugged the snare like a fishing line. The polyp came closer, into full view.

"Whoa! That's a mean mother!" Karl hooted. "I'm telling you, it's dangerous. Leave it and get the heck out of there!"

I remained silent. The position was ideal. The colon was not moving. There was full insufflation; the colon was well distended. I watched, astonished and grateful.

"We're in good position," I croaked, suppressing my surprise.

"Whoa! Smooth!" Karl said. "Smooth moves, man! Great technique!"

I shrugged, projecting nonchalance.

"Close snare," I ordered.

Penny tightened the snare and the polyp swelled up and turned purple. A few beads of blood dripped off.

"Whoa! It's going to bleed! Stop!" Karl yelped.

"No! Cut it!" I insisted. My heart was beating like a drum.

Penny closed the snare completely. It sliced through the stalk and the polyp immediately slumped over. A trickle of blood crept from the stalk. My heart pounded and my head throbbed painfully. For a minute, there was utter silence in the room.

"Amazing!" Penny whispered.

It was perfect. The stump was tiny and pink, and the polyp had fallen on its side like a tree. There was no further bleeding. We all stared at the screen in awe.

"Well, butter my butt and call me a biscuit!" Karl declared.

"That looks good," I allowed. My voice was raspy.

"Good? Man, that was *awesome!*" Karl enthused. "That was the best damn polypectomy I have ever seen!"

My mouth was so dry that I just nodded.

"Look at you, man! Cool as ice!" Karl whooped.

The only parts of me that weren't shaking were my shoulders, so I shrugged.

"*Iceman!* You're a dang iceman!" Karl said, reverently.

A trickle of blood emerged from the stump. I turned to Penny.

"Adrenaline!" I whispered.

I injected adrenaline into the stump again. The bleeding stopped. We waited anxiously.

No more bleeding.

My heart slowed down and I swallowed again.

"That was awesome," Karl said, "Hey, Dell Clawsom is still waiting. He doesn't like to be kept waiting."

Karl walked out.

"Penny, I'm going to put the snare back in to grab the polyp that we just cut. It's way too big to suck out through the scope," I said.

"Do you think we need any more adrenaline?" Penny asked.

"We need to watch for bleeding. She could still bleed."

I re-introduced the snare. Before I could grasp the polyp, the tip of the snare jabbed the stump, and it started spurting. The screen rapidly turned crimson. My mouth dried out completely and my heart raced.

"Doctor! It's bleeding! Bleeding a lot!" Penny shrieked.

"I know. Remove the snare! Give me more adrenaline, now!"

We furiously exchanged the snare for the adrenaline injector.

"Get ready to push the needle out! I need to inject the stump while I can still see it!"

Blood gushed out of the stump. Within seconds, it was covered up.

"Gwen was right, her mother is an easy bleeder," Penny said.

I flushed with water but the bleeding was profuse.

"I can't see anything," Penny said. "How do you know where to inject?"

"I'll have to go blind," I said grimly. I advanced the needle towards my last sighting of the stump.

"Needle out!" I ordered. Penny pushed the tip of the needle out. I thrust it into my target.

"One cc now," I instructed. I saw the lining swell up with the injection.

I removed the needle and reinserted it a few millimeters to the right.

"Inject again, one more cc," I said.

"Doc, I'm out of adrenaline."

"What? You're out of adrenaline?" I was shocked.

"That's why I was asking if you needed any more."

"Of course I need adrenaline!" I shouted. "What were you thinking?"

"I only brought one syringe and I lost some of it when I was flushing the injection catheter."

I bit my lip.

"What more could possibly go wrong?" I howled.

"I'm so sorry!" Penny wailed.

I flushed with water. I couldn't see anything. There was blood everywhere.

"Should I run down to the pharmacy and get some more adrenaline?"

"No, we don't have time. Just draw up ten cc of saline right now, stat!"

"I left the sterile saline in the pharmacy too!" Penny cried. "I'm so sorry! I'm so sorry!"

"Then draw up ten cc of saline from the patient's IV bag!"

She did as ordered.

"Now we're going to inject saline into the stump. Get ready."

Penny attached the syringe of saline to the injection needle.

"So we're going to inject saline instead of adrenaline?"

"Yes. It's not perfect but it will put pressure on the stump just long enough for me to put the clip."

I guessed the location of the stump and injected saline repeatedly in that area. Slowly, the bleeding slowed down and I was able to see the stump again. Drops of blood kept forming and dripping.

"The clip! *Now!* Give me the clip!" I shrieked.

Penny was a blur. She tore open the package, pulled out the clip forceps, straightened it out, and slid it smoothly into the scope. It popped out the other end and appeared on the screen.

"Excellent! Open the clip! I'm in a good position!" I cried.

She opened the jaws of the clip. I hovered right above the dripping stump.

"Close! Close hard!" I ordered.

Penny slammed the clip shut. The clip pinched the tissue at an angle and the dripping stopped immediately.

We watched the screen anxiously. The stump turned pale. I reintroduced the injection forceps and waited.

"I'm injecting one more time, as a precaution. Give me another two cc of saline now," I said.

I injected both sides of the clip. I washed the area with water. The stump remained dry. I exchanged the injector for the snare forceps and grabbed the cut polyp with it, and dragged it out. I withdrew the endoscope completely and we both exhaled.

"Oh, my goodness!" Penny gasped, "Just look at the size of that polyp!"

Emily moaned and passed a large blood clot.

"Oh no!" Penny wailed, "She's bleeding again! She's bleeding!"

As if to confirm her worst fears, the patient obligingly passed another, even larger, clot.

"What are we going to *do*, Doctor?"

I wasn't sure.

"Do you want me to get some O negative blood?"

I hesitated.

"It didn't look like that much bleeding. Maybe that's just old blood."

"It looked red, Doctor."

"Well, she only stopped bleeding a few minutes ago. Could be old stuff."

"So you're sure there's nothing to worry about?"

I hesitated.

"Let's look again."

I wiped the endoscope and re-inserted it. I reached the site and washed it.

It was not bleeding.

"It's not bleeding," I said, trying to sound confident.

I waited for a few minutes. It did not bleed.

"Not bleeding but I want to be safe. Give me another metal clip."

Penny had it ready, and handed it to me quickly. I passed it through the endoscope and clipped the stump at right angles to the first clip.

"I see the base of the polyp and I've put a second metal clip there," I explained.

"Each clip costs the hospital three hundred dollars," Penny said.

"ICU admission costs far more," I countered.

Penny nodded.

"That should hold it nicely," I said, keeping my voice steady.

"We sure don't want her bleeding to death," Penny declared. "She scared the holy crap out of me, Doc. Pardon my French."

I removed the endoscope for the second time and wiped it down again. I handed it to Penny.

"You look a little shaken," Penny said. "I guess that kind of scared the crap out of you, too, huh?"

I shrugged and removed my mask and gown.

"No, no. Done it before in Houston and London," I croaked.

"But not in Hotspur," Penny beamed. "I bet you've never done anything like this before!"

"I'm going to my office to write my operative note," I said, keeping my voice steady. My legs were weak and I desperately needed coffee and fluids.

"Yes, Doctor. Good job!" Penny sang out.

I nodded and walked out stiffly, turning the lights on as I left. Out of Penny's sight, I staggered across the corridor quickly. I steadied myself on the doorframe before entering the clinic. I overheard Karl talking to the office staff.

"There he was, that little dude, cool as ice, and he just chopped off that humongous polyp like it was *nothing!*" he recounted incredulously.

I was grateful that the room had been dark.

"Man, he was cool as ice! Didn't even break a sweat!"

I waited for the pounding on my chest to slow down and the moisture to return to my mouth. I tested my voice before I sauntered in.

"There he is!" Karl announced, "There he is! The man of the hour! Mr. Cool Hand Luke! Man, that was something else! You've got some freaking nerve!"

"Some nerve? About what?" I feigned ignorance.

"About what? About that monster polyp, that's what!"

I nodded, as if trying to remember the incident.

"Oh, that polyp? Yeah, that was kind of a big polyp," I acknowledged.

"*Kind of?* It was a freaking mother of a polyp!" Karl thundered. "A freaking mother!"

"Dr. Becker, language!" Tracy scolded.

"You took a little time to wind up after I left," Karl noted, "Did you have any problems?"

I shrugged and sauntered over to the coffee machine and helped myself. Karl wouldn't find out the details for another thirty minutes, so I basked in the admiring gazes of Tracy, Ginger, Kendra, and two patients checking in at the window. I choked down a mug of hot, black liquid and took a deep breath.

"Yeah. Little bit of bleeding, yeah. Nothing much," I declared, airily. "The ones I did in Houston and London, you should have seen *those*. This was nothing. Didn't stress me at all."

CHAPTER 2

A SMALL FAVOR

I drained my coffee and set it down.

"Dell Clawsom said he couldn't wait. He left," Tracy said.

"What?" I was immediately deflated.

"He said he'll call you later," Tracy said.

"I was delayed because that was a complicated procedure," I huffed.

"I told him that," Tracy said, "but he said he had to go. He had something to do in his hangar."

"His hangar?"

"Yes. He owns the Warbird Museum. He's got a lot of planes."

"That's right. I had forgotten."

Tracy was admiring a tall silver cylinder.

"Have you seen this, Dr. Mathur? The girls got it for Dr. Becker, to welcome him back."

It was a large insulated, stainless steel coffee mug, adorned with a stethoscope curling around a background of stars and stripes. The words 'Our Hero' had been engraved in glittering red letters. Tracy held it high and rotated it proudly.

"Very nice," I said, without much enthusiasm.

"Do you have one?" Tracy asked.

"No," I replied.

"Oh. The girls must have forgotten to get you one. Sorry."

"That's okay. I don't need one."

"But you like to have coffee."

"I'm perfectly fine with a regular mug or a styrofoam cup."

"I'll remind the girls that they need to order one for you."

"I really don't care."

"It's not fair. This nice, big, beautiful cup for Dr. Becker, and nothing for you."

Tracy watched me for my reaction.

"It's fine," I lied, "I don't care. I'm going to my office."

When I got to my office the phone was ringing. It was my wife, Maya.

"I have a favor to ask," she said.

"Go ahead."

Maya hesitated.

"You know that seamstress we use? The one who altered your interview suit?"

"Yes. Valerie Berlinghieri. I remember her."

"She called me at home. Said she has a problem. Her husband swallowed a battery."

"A battery?"

"Yes. A small battery. He was changing his car key battery and dropped it in his food. Then he ate the food and felt something stick but it had gone down before he could do anything about it."

"Was it a disc battery?"

"I don't know."

"I'll call her and find out. If it's a disc battery, then we need to get it out. It can get stuck and cause serious problems."

Maya gave me Valerie's number. Minutes later, I was talking to her.

"I'm so sorry to bother you, Dr. Mathur, but my little Rico just swallowed one of those flat little batteries. I didn't know what to do so I asked Dr. Becker, his regular doctor."

"What did Dr. Becker say?" I asked. The words *Our Hero* flashed in front of me. I blocked them out.

"He said, it's a big deal, we need to get him to a specialist in Abilene."

"Okay, send him to Abilene."

Valerie paused.

"But *you're* a specialist, aren't you? You're the kind of specialist we would have to see in Abilene. So I asked myself, Valerie, why are you going to take poor little Rico all the way to Abilene when you've got a wonderful little specialist right here in Hotspur?"

"A *little* specialist?"

"Yes," Valerie went on, with relentless enthusiasm. "Our own little specialist right here. *You* can get that dad gum battery out of my little Rico, can't you? The hospital bought you that nice scope thingy."

"Thingy? It's an endoscope."

"That sounds right. Endoscope. Can't you go down his mouth and pull it out? That way we don't have to go to Abilene. We can stay right here and get treated."

"Well, it can be tricky," I said. I had just come out of a crisis, and was still rattled.

"You're a specialist! We trust you!" Valerie pleaded.

I dismissed my hesitation. I was keen to use the new endoscope, and I didn't have any patients in the clinic.

"Yes, we have an upper endoscope," I answered. "I can handle it."

"Can I bring him right over?" Valerie asked. "We live in the country, Horsethieves Gulch. Fifteen minutes, tops."

"Yes. Go ahead. I have some in-patients to see in the hospital but I should be done by the time you get here. Come over right away. We'll get him up to the OR and pull that battery out of his food pipe before it gets into his stomach."

Simon called an hour later. He was British, and I enjoyed hearing his accent. It reminded me of my years in London.

"Your patient is finally on his way in, Dr. Mathur. He's coming by ambulance," he said.

"By ambulance? For a swallowed battery?"

"He can't breathe, sir."

"Did the battery go into his airway?"

"No, sir. He has severe sleep apnea. He's three hundred and seventy-two pounds."

"What? I didn't know that! She called him 'my little Rico' just now!"

"He's a big boy, sir."

"This complicates things!"

"He's choking on his own saliva. Took four lads to load him into the ambulance! He's a bloody mess, sir."

My mouth dried up for the second time that morning.

"I think he should go to Abilene," I said.

"I agree. But you already accepted him and this is the nearest ER. So we have to see him, sir. Those are the rules."

I groaned. My heart sank; I had walked into another crisis.

"We'll never be able to transfer him! No one will accept him, I know. I shouldn't have offered to help," I moaned.

Simon was not sympathetic.

"Well, you are a specialist, Dr. Mathur. It's your subject."

"Yes, but he's so big! Based upon that weight, he must have severe sleep apnea. There's no anesthesiologist here, no ICU or ventilator, in fact, no backup whatsoever. I don't know what I can do for this man."

"They expect you to remove the battery, sir."

"Call Penny and have her bring the endoscopy cart and monitor to the ER. We may have to scope him right there."

"Don't you want to take him to the Operating Room, sir?"

"Our OR table can't take anyone over three hundred and fifty pounds. It could collapse. The one in the ER might be able to handle him. Anyway, it's going to be difficult to get him up to the second floor, and the equipment here isn't working, anyway."

"Then ER it is. I'll call Penny. Thank you, sir."

Rico Berlinghieri was enormous. His face was as large as a dinner plate, red and bloated. His eyes were swollen shut and a full-sized plastic facemask squeezed his nose, mouth and cheeks into a fleshy donut. He wheezed loudly and rasped as oxygen whistled around him. He squirmed and tugged at the tubes that tethered him to an oxygen cylinder. Three burly paramedics unlocked him from their stretcher and rolled him over onto the ER table. The ER table lurched, rocked, but remained intact.

"Leave him on his left side, not flat on his back," I ordered.

A tall, slim woman in a beehive hairdo and enormous square glasses rushed forward. She spoke in a hoarse voice.

"Thank you for seeing my little Rico," Valerie said. "It all happened so fast! I'm so sorry, I'm still in my bathrobe!"

She wore a fluffy pink bathrobe with matching slippers. There were small round burn marks on her robes. She had traces of purple make-up on her eyes and cheeks.

"My little Rico was changing my car key battery. He put it down on his breakfast plate and it must have fallen into his eggs."

"So there's food in his stomach?" I said, alarmed.

"Just a little. He had a little breakfast. Is that a problem?"

I groaned.

"Yes. That makes it more difficult. What else did he have?"

"Let me see. Really, just the usual. Eggs, bacon, hash browns, coffee, and toast. Maybe a teeny bite of a brownie with his coffee."

"That means there's a lot of food in his stomach. I hope the battery is still in his food pipe, it's going to be very difficult to get it out if it falls into his stomach."

"Can't swallow," Rico gurgled, and started spitting. Simon slid a plastic basin under his mouth and gave him paper towels. Rico heaved and spat out a fistful of foamy spittle. Valerie rushed to his side and rubbed his forehead.

"My *poor* little Rico! He can't swallow! Doctor, please, please help him!"

I snatched up the clipboard and scanned the paramedic's notes.

"So he's fifty-seven years old, retired, an ex-smoker, has high blood pressure and diabetes and thyroid problems. What else? Any surgeries?"

"Oh, I forgot. Bypass surgery and heart stents."

"When was the bypass? How many vessels?"

"Three-way bypass five years ago. Five stents, last two went in a year ago."

I examined him quickly.

"His heart sounds are muffled by his lungs. He's wheezing pretty badly. What are these scars on his belly?" I asked.

"Oh, I forgot. It's been so long. He had some intestine cut out because it was twisted. But that was years ago."

"Does he have chest pain?"

"Only when he walks to the mailbox."

"How far is that? How many steps?"

"Maybe thirty or forty."

"Shortness of breath?"

"When he walks a few steps."

"Does he snore?"

Rico snorted. Valerie smiled indulgently.

"Like a freight train, Doctor. Luckily we live out in the country. He would keep the whole street awake if he lived here, I reckon," she said.

"Simon, please start an IV and get labs. I want a CBC, CMP and TSH and an EKG. Check his oxygen saturation and keep him on the face mask at forty percent. Call Abilene and tell them we have an urgent transfer," I said.

"Transfer? You're not going to treat him here?" Valerie was taken aback.

"No. He's too complicated. We don't have anesthesia and we don't have ICU backup. I can't sedate him safely. Our sedating medicine might stop his breathing completely. He already has serious heart and lung problems."

"But you said you could scope him!" Valerie complained.

"I can definitely scope him, but we need a different specialist called an anesthesiologist, to protect his heart and lungs."

"Do we not have one?" Valerie asked.

"No. He needs to go to Abilene."

"They won't take him! Doc, we don't have insurance!" Valerie wailed.

"Doesn't matter. He has an emergency. They have to take him."

Valerie shook her head.

"Your wife said you were a specialist. I thought *you* could take care of him."

"I can do the endoscopy, but I need someone else to sedate him, and look after his breathing while I do my job. Otherwise, he's going to fight me when I put the scope in his mouth"

"Give him some medicine, my sweet little Rico won't fight you."

"He's a big boy and he has severe sleep apnea. Such patients are at high risk for anesthesia. He may stop breathing or suck food into his lungs. It's too dangerous!"

Valerie put her hands on her hips and shook her head in disbelief

"So you won't do *anything* for him?" Valerie wondered, her voice quivering. "You're just going to give up? Why won't you help him?"

"Of course we're going to help him! Let me explain. First, he's over three hundred pounds, right?"

"Three hundred and seventy-two."

"Exactly. So that's very high risk right there. Second, he has heart and lung disease. So he's at even greater risk if we sedate him for the test and reduce his oxygen level. He could have a heart attack or stroke!"

Valerie gazed back at me, unfazed. I went on.

"Finally, he has had abdominal surgery. If that small battery gets into his stomach then it will be incredibly difficult to get it out with all the food there. While we're messing around in his stomach, he could throw up and the food could get sucked into his lungs."

"What if you can't get it out of his stomach?" Valerie asked.

"If the battery leaves the stomach and gets into his intestine, it will probably get stuck."

"Why would it get stuck in his intestine?"

"Because he's had surgery on his intestine. You just told me. That means there will be some scarring and narrowing so the battery is likely to get stuck if it leaves the stomach."

"It's just a little battery! I can't believe it's causing all these problems!"

"That's the problem. Because it's a small battery, the two ends are close to each other and both ends will be touching his tissue. That allows an electric current to pass and it burns the tissue. Also the battery can get very hot."

"So it could burn a hole in his stomach or intestine?"

"Possibly."

"Then what do we do if he burns a hole?"

"Then he's definitely going to need an operation. You see, it's too risky! He needs to go to Abilene right away!"

Valerie thought for a minute. She crossed her arms and glared.

"So you're not even going to *try?*"

"No. It's too risky."

"Because we don't have insurance?"

"No, because it's too risky."

"But you're a specialist!"

I didn't want to hear that word again. I spoke slowly.

"Yes, but I need other specialists to back me up. I can't do everything on my own."

Valerie turned to Rico. Rico gagged and shook his head. He struggled to sit up.

"Doc, Doc," he sputtered, "I can't go on like this, Doc. Just do it. Do the best you can!"

Rico pushed himself up and tried to grab my wrist.

"For God's sake, do it! I've never had so much pain in my life!" he gasped.

"Rico, it's too risky!" I countered

"Can't go on, Doc! That dang battery's burning me up like fire!"

I hesitated. It was an emergency, and it would be at least an hour before

I could get him seen in Abilene. *If* I could get anyone to even accept him.

"Please, Doc! Do it! Just do it, we don't got the time to go nowhere else!" Rico pleaded.

Penny flung open the door and heaved the endoscopy cart inside. The small monitor rocked and the scope rattled against the metal frame. I helped her roll the cart into a corner and locked the wheels.

"Gee, thanks, Doctor," Penny said, cheerfully. "So let's get this show on the road! You're the man! The second big case of the day!"

She sensed the tension.

"What's the matter?"

"He's too complicated. We need to send him to Abilene."

"But you're a specialist!" she sang out.

I groaned.

"Anyway, they won't take him," Penny said. Simon nodded.

"I called the Abilene ER on your polyp patient. They said, you can't transfer to a higher level of care because you already are a specialist," he said.

"But I need someone to look after this man's airway! I can do the scope but what if he stops breathing or sucks stomach contents into his lungs after I sedate him?"

"Dr. Becker said you need to explain that to the gastroenterologist there, Dr. Wegener."

"Then get Dr. Wegener on the line."

"He's tied up in a case right now. He's busy."

"When will he call me back?"

"The ER didn't know. Whenever he's done and gets your message, I guess."

I looked at Rico. His vital signs were stable. His blood pressure was holding. His heart rate was rapid, but that was to be expected. His oxygen saturation was ninety percent, which was borderline.

"If we wait too long, the battery will drop into the stomach," I said.

"We don't want that," Valerie declared.

"If I can just go into the food pipe and grab the battery very quickly and get it out, it just might work," I said.

"You can do it, Doc!" Valerie enthused. Rico nodded.

Simon shook his head and pretended to slit his throat with his finger.

"I bet he can handle your little surgery, Doc, he's a mean son-of-a-gun," Valerie said. "But if we wait and he needs major surgery, he won't make it."

I nodded. Simon stepped forward.

"He could die after major surgery, sir. What if we just wait and let the battery come out on its own, sir? I question you only because the risks are so high," Simon said.

"If the battery stays in his food pipe, it will burn a hole there. If it gets into his stomach, we will lose it in the food there. If it gets into his intestine, it will get stuck there and Rico will need an operation to cut it out," I said.

The door was thrown open and Dr. Becker stormed inside. He wore biking shorts and shirt and brandished his personalized coffee cup.

"Why the heck are you seeing my patient?" he stormed.

"Your patient?" I asked.

"Yes, my patient! I told Penny!"

I turned to Penny. She shrugged.

"I was about to tell you. I forgot. Sorry," she said, blithely.

"His wife called Maya, and Maya called me," I explained.

Karl glared at Valerie, who looked away and said nothing.

"Are you crazy?" Karl thundered. "Are you completely nuts?"

"What do you mean?" I stammered.

"Are you seriously planning to do an upper endoscopy on this sorry specimen?"

"I was thinking about it, yes," I admitted.

Karl dropped his jaw dramatically. He waved his steel coffee cup in astonishment.

"You are crazier than I thought! Taking out a polyp on a stable patient is a different matter. Look at him! Rico has severe sleep apnea! Are you going to sedate him? He's going to quit breathing! He'll have a cardiac arrest and die right in front of you before you can say *oh crap*!"

My apprehension turned to dread.

"You see how big he is? Do you know how much medicine he's going to take?" Dr. Becker hooted.

"I was planning to use small doses of midazolam," I said.

"Midazolam? You can hit him with ten or twelve or even fifteen, it won't even touch him!"

"Maybe use a little propofol?"

"He's eaten his usual breakfast, which is probably three times what everyone else eats. So you'll have to go there and drag your little net through the mass of food in his belly."

"If I can just get into the esophagus and grab it out of there before it drops into the stomach, I'll be okay," I ventured.

"I called my buddy, Marty Wegener, in Abilene. He's in the gastro group there. He refused to take Rico. Refused! Said he was too high risk, said to ship him to Dallas."

"Yes, great," I said, sensing an escape. "Let's ship him to Dallas!"

"What do you think I've been doing, Einstein? I've been calling Dallas. No one wants him," Karl said, "No one. Not St. Jo, not Mercy, not even Plainview Peaks Hospital."

"So what do we do?" I asked.

Karl took a long and thoughtful draught of coffee.

"Your coffee cup says, *Our Hero*! That's so sweet!" Penny applauded. Karl ignored her.

"I told that old fart Wegener that you were here, that you were a trained gastro doc, and he says, well, great, let Mathur deal with it then, he's a specialist same as me, and hangs up! Can you believe that? Hangs up on *me!*"

Karl picked up the ER chart and glanced at it.

"Thanks for trying," I said.

Karl was seething.

"I can't believe the jerk hung up on me. But I'm just a country boy, small town doc who knows diddly-squat about anything."

"What are you saying?"

"All I'm saying is that if *you*, being a specialist the same as he is, if *you* were to call him and ask for his help, I reckon he'll say okay. Maybe he just wants us to grovel a little."

I hated the idea, but I was cornered.

"I don't mind calling him. Anyway, it'll be nice to meet other gastroenterologists in the area."

Dr. Becker laughed.

"You obviously don't know Dr. Wegener. He can be a royal pain. You're going to have to really grovel, okay?"

"Really grovel?" I repeated, taken aback.

"Yes. Really grovel. Eat dirt. Beg him. Kiss his hand."

"Why?"

"That's just his personality, man. He's the perfect gastroenterologist because he truly is nothing but an asshole!"

I didn't want to call Dr. Wegener.

"So I need to call this Dr. Wegener and plead with him?"

"Einstein, I've done the pleading! You need to beg and grovel for his help. Be pitiful. Effing pathetic!"

"I don't like doing that," I said, feeling angry and resentful.

"Put on your big-boy panties and deal with it! You may be asking him for a job, right? I mean you're the same kind of specialist but you're stuck in this hick town, in the last year of your contract, fixing to get the heck out of here! So be real nice to him, lick his hand, or lick whatever, bow down, kiss his feet, whatever. Specialists will listen to other specialists more than to lowly family docs."

I stared at Karl. He was actually enjoying this.

"Can *you* call him again? This is your patient, really," I said, weakly.

Karl snatched up the chart and scanned it.

"Oh, really? *My* patient? I'm so sorry, Excellency, it seems they put *you* down as the doctor. *You* accepted him. So it's *your* ass on the line! Deal with it," he snapped. He tossed the chart back to Simon, who fumbled and dropped it on the floor. It came apart, and Simon scrambled to gather the pages.

Karl spun around and shot out, and slammed the door behind him.

Penny, Simon and I gazed at each other in shock and confusion. Valerie gaped at us and flung both arms around Rico, who gurgled and retched even louder.

"I'm sorry, I'm so sorry!" Valerie cried. "I got you into this. I just wanted someone to help my little Rico. No one else wants to touch him!"

Simon looked at the scrambled chart and shook his head.

"No good deed goes unpunished," he said.

CHAPTER 3

THE SPECIALIST TAKES CHARGE

"So what do we do now?" Penny asked.

I looked at Simon for guidance. Simon dramatically sliced his finger across his neck again.

"Why is it so urgent to get the battery out?" he asked. "It's just a little button battery, sir."

"It's a fifteen millimeter button battery. It gets stuck in the food pipe and leaks chemicals. An electric current flows around it through the tissues. The chemicals and electricity burn the tissue and can punch a hole through it!"

"Are you serious? Could that really happen?" Simon gaped.

"Yes," I said. "The battery could also get very hot, produce poisonous gas and even explode."

"What? Doctor, I didn't know that!" Valerie cried.

"Penny, get Mr. Berlinghieri to sign a consent for the procedure. Simon, get me two ten milligram vials of midazolam and one hundred milligrams of propofol and three vials of romazicon from the pharmacy!" I ordered.

Simon broke out of his trance. He sat the chart aside and I scribbled the order for the medicines. He grabbed it and rushed off to the pharmacy.

"Rico, I need you to understand there are serious risks of this procedure. You could choke on your fluids, the food that you ate earlier, or even the battery. Those things could all get sucked into your lungs. Also you could have a heart attack or stop breathing due to the medicines we give you to put you to sleep."

Rico shuddered. Valerie stiffened.

"There's also the risk of a drug reaction and infection and other fatal complications. In other words, you could die from this procedure. Do you want to proceed? Do you consent to this procedure?" I asked.

Rico nodded and signed the form. Valerie co-signed, kissed his forehead, and stepped back.

"Wait by the Coke machine, sweetheart," Penny said. Valerie nodded and disappeared. She looked badly shaken and on the verge of tears.

I slipped on a protective gown and face shield. Penny checked the endoscope and handed me gloves and shoe-covers.

"Rico, I'm going to place this little bite-block between your teeth," she said.

"Huh?"

"It's a piece of plastic with a hole in it so we can protect your teeth from the scope and protect the scope from your teeth. The doctor will push the scope in through that little hole."

Rico nodded. Penny strapped it in place. She replaced the facemask.

Simon reappeared with the vials.

"Draw up ten milligrams of the midazolam and one vial of romazicon," I said.

"Why the romazicon?" Penny asked.

"It's the antidote for midazolam. In case I give too much midazolam, I can reverse it with romazicon."

"That's perfect!"

"To a point. Once I reverse the sedation, I can't start again. So I really don't want to use it if I can help it."

"Then just give him very little," Penny suggested.

"I can't do that. He's a big boy, and he's going to need a lot. But if I give him just a little too much, he could stop breathing completely."

"Then what?"

"Then I'll have to give him the antidote and abort everything," I said.

"I guess you're doing this because you've done this many times in Houston and London, right?" Penny asked.

"Yes."

"Like the big polyp you just took out, right?"

"Right."

Penny hesitated.

"Because you're a specialist, right?"

I nodded.

"Not because you don't want to beg the specialist in Abilene or Dallas to take over?"

"I don't mind begging. Fact is, we just don't have the time. The battery starts causing damage in two hours. Then after it burns the food pipe it will drop into the stomach full of food and we'll never get it out."

A thought struck me.

"Simon, call CA in hospital maintenance. Tell him I want the biggest magnet he can find," I said.

"They don't have magnets in maintenance," Simon said.

"Tell him to open any electric motor and pull out the permanent magnet inside, and bring it up here right away."

Simon relayed the message. To my relief, CA did not question my order.

"So is a disc battery magnetisable, sir?" Simon asked.

"Yes. It has a stainless steel jacket. I used a magnet once in London."

"In London?"

"Yes. A disc battery had dropped into a pool of food and I managed to drag it out with a magnet," I said.

"But this isn't London or Houston, and we don't have special magnets," Simon added, helpfully.

"Thank you for reminding me. I had almost forgotten," I snapped.

Simon was immediately contrite.

"My apologies, sir. I was merely alluding to the fact that you have extensive experience in these matters."

"No, I don't think you were. That's okay. When CA brings the magnet, wrap it in a pillow case."

Simon nodded.

"Okay, the scope is ready," Penny announced.

"Turn the lights down and I'm going to give Rico two-point-five milligrams of midazolam."

I injected the midazolam and we waited two minutes. Rico still gazed at me, wide-eyed and fearful.

"No effect with two-point-five. I'm going to give another one-point-five of midazolam."

We waited another two minutes. Rico's eyelids began to flutter, but he fought the medicine and stayed awake.

"He's still awake. I'm giving him another milligram."

As we watched, Rico's eyelids drooped and his breathing slowed down.

"His oxygen saturation's dropping, sir!" Simon called out.

"I expected that. Give me the scope. He'll wake up a bit when I put this in his mouth."

I placed the tip of the endoscope gingerly in Rico's mouth. He coughed and reared up. I withdrew hastily.

"Penny, give him another milligram. Actually, make that one-point-five milligrams."

Penny looked dubious. The phone started ringing.

"Sir, his oxygen is dropping. He started at ninety-one percent and now he's eighty-eight percent. Are you sure you want to give more midazolam?"

"We need to do this. Give the midazolam."

"Are you sure, sir?" she persisted.

I was irritated, but held back.

"Yes," I said. "Simon! Please answer the phone."

Simon snatched it up.

"Hotspur Hospital ER, Simon Godwyn RN speaking, how can I help you?"

Simon listened for a minute and covered the mouthpiece.

"It's the Abilene Hospital. They're getting Dr. Wegener on the phone," he said.

I took the phone and waited.

"Your call is very important for us. Please continue to hold," the recording said. I looked at Rico.

"Rico looks pretty awake," I declared.

Simon coughed and weighed in.

"That's a total of five already in and another one-and-half will make it six point five milligrams of midazolam, sir. That's a pretty stiff dose, sir."

I nodded.

"He's a big boy. He may even need a little more. Let's see."

I continued to hold. I listened to the Four Seasons by Vivaldi.

"Your call is very important to us. Please continue to hold."

Rico's eyes drooped. His head slumped.

"He's getting there! He might be sleepy enough for me to get started!" I said. We all watched Rico carefully.

"Your call is very important to us. Please continue to hold."

We watched Rico for two minutes. Instead of sleeping, he became more restive and started moving around.

"He's not going to sleep, Doctor," Penny said.

"I agree. He's going to need some more sedation. Simon, draw up another milligram."

"Not to conflict with your orders, sir, but is that wise? He looks pretty sleepy to me," Simon said.

"Simon, put this call on speaker. I'll push the midazolam, you just listen and give me the phone when Dr. Wegener comes on."

Simon looked uncomfortable. He took over the phone.

"If he stops breathing, it's going to be very difficult to put a tube in his airway," he warned.

"I understand your concern, Simon. I'm watching him closely."

"Your call is very important to us. Please continue to hold."

I gave Rico another milligram of midazolam. Within seconds, an alarm screamed.

"Holy crap! Oxygen's fallen to eighty-five percent!" Penny cried.

The door burst open again and Kurt stood at the threshold.

"What? You're actually doing it?" he bellowed, "Are you totally nuts?"

"The oxygen's dropped to eighty-five percent," Simon echoed.

"Come here and give him a jaw thrust," I ordered.

"Dang! Eighty-five's pretty dang low, man!" Kurt echoed.

Rico needed stimulation. There was no choice. I placed the tip of the scope in Rico's mouth and slid it over the tongue and past the vocal cords in a single movement. Rico shuddered and bucked. Simon jumped and held him down. Penny replaced the oxygen mask and clamped it tightly over his face.

"Whoa! You're in the esophagus now, ace!" Kurt said.

"You woke him up! Sats now ninety percent!" Simon added.

"Your call is very important to us. Please continue to hold."

"Are you holding on Wegener?" Karl asked.

"Yes. We were on hold so long I put it on speakerphone. Hang it up now."

I pushed down a little to the middle of the food pipe. Karl peered at the screen.

The phone rang again. Simon grabbed it and listened. He turned to me.

"They've paged Dr. Wegener again. They want us to keep holding," he said, shaking his head.

"Forget it. Hang up. I need you here."

"But what about transferring him to Abilene?"

"At this point he's more likely to stop breathing and die!" I snapped.

"But we need Dr. Wegener to accept the patient," Simon pointed out.

I thought quickly.

"Okay, let's hold on for five minutes. Then hang up and don't answer it again."

"Whoa! Sounds like Mr. Cool Hand Luke is getting pissed off," Karl chuckled.

"He made me wait on the line and now he's making me wait again," I complained.

"Life's not fair, Einstein. Didn't you know that? I told you, you got to kiss his ass!"

I inflated gas in the food pipe and advanced the tip slowly. Karl peered at the screen.

"So where is it? Where's the dang battery?" he questioned

"It's usually at the lower end of the food pipe, because there's a natural narrowing there," I said, struggling to sound calm. Rico heaved and moved his head. I washed and suctioned and inflated gas.

No battery.

"Well, you got his oxygen back up, ace!" Karl said, "But maybe you're all wrong about the battery."

"Our portable X-ray machine is down, and we can't get him onto X-ray so I can't really see where the battery is right now," I explained.

I pushed further down to the lower end of the food pipe. There was a food plug blocking the opening. I washed and suctioned again, turning the jet of water from side to side. The viscous material was whittled away. The battery was there, jammed diagonally like a no-smoking sign, glittering yellow with bile.

"There she is!" Kurt yelled, "You were right! There she be! Man oh man, it's already burned up the dang lining."

"The lining where the battery is stuck looks chalky white," Penny observed.

"Your call is very important to us. Please continue to hold."

"The lining turns white and swells up because of the electric current and the leakage of chemicals," I said, forcing my voice to remain steady. I felt humbled by the inattention from Abilene.

I inflated carbon dioxide gas and stretched the food pipe wide open. The lining stretched a little but the battery remained stuck.

"It's fixed to the lining! That's a bad sign," I groaned.

"A bad sign? Why?" Penny asked.

"Because it's generating enough heat to sear the tissue all around the rim."

"So the rim has burnt into the lining?"

"Exactly. We have to tear it off the lining. Give me a Roth net."

Penny peeled one open and handed me the tip. I fed it in and saw it reappear on the screen.

"Your call is very important to us. Please continue …"

"Hang it up!" I snarled.

"Temper, temper," Karl chided.

I used the tip of the device to try to dislodge the battery, but the tip kept sliding off the smooth surface.

"Do you want to try something else?" Karl asked. "You got any other toys?"

"No. I'm going to push harder."

It didn't work. Frustrated, I advanced the scope and slammed it against the battery.

"Watch out! Don't tear it off and drop it into the stomach!" Penny warned.

I pulled back to survey the results. The battery had been partly torn off.

"The lining is bleeding, Doctor!"

"Yes, but we may have an opportunity. I'm going to advance the net through that opening."

The phone rang again. Simon looked at me. I shrugged and returned to the procedure. Simon answered the phone and was put on hold.

"Open the net," I ordered. "Don't put the phone on speaker, it's distracting. He's not going to answer anyway."

Penny tried to open the Roth net. On the screen, the tip shuddered and twisted, but the net did not emerge.

"It won't open, Doctor. It's jammed."

"Pull it back, straighten it out and try again."

Penny struggled.

"It's not working, Doctor."

"Push harder!"

"I haven't done this before. I don't want to break it, Doctor."

Kurt set down his coffee mug and grabbed the handle of the net forceps.

"Let me do this," he said. He pushed hard.

The net burst out and hit the battery like a ram, and ripped it off completely. There was a gush of blood and bile and the battery disappeared. Rico retched and flailed. His foot caught Simon in the groin and Simon was thrown against the sink. The phone fell out of his hand.

"See? That got it loose!" Karl said, triumphantly, and handed the forceps back to Penny.

I flushed desperately with water. *I need to grab that battery before it drops into the stomach!* The battery glinted through the swirling fluids.

"I see the battery. Go get it, ace!" Karl enthused, waving his mug.

Rico retched again and there was a tidal wave of yellow and green frothy stomach contents. It shot up to his mouth and he coughed violently. Vomitus flooded his facemask. I yanked the endoscope out.

"Raise up the head end of the bed! Don't let that get into his lungs!" I cried. "Throw away that face mask! Get him a new one!"

We rushed to stabilize Rico, but it was too late for the battery. After I re-inserted the scope and suctioned the food pipe dry, it had vanished. Rico was waking up rapidly so I removed the scope again and laid it down on the cart.

"Crap!" Penny said, glumly, "Crappity crap crap! Battery's gone!"

"Have we lost the battery?" Simon asked.

"Yeah, it's in the stomach now," Karl said. "But your Royal Physician Dr. Mathur can get it out. You know why? Because he's a *specialist*."

He turned to leave.

"Hey, y'all! Seen my new coffee mug? The office staff had it made specially for me," he said. I glimpsed the steel cylinder with shiny letters that spelled *Our Hero*.

"Oh, very nice!" Simon enthused. I said nothing.

"Hey, Einstein, I almost forgot. You got another patient waiting in the clinic. Won't see me. Says she only wants to see *the specialist*."

"Thanks for your help, Karl."

"Not much help. Knocked the dang thing into the stomach. Whatever. I got to go see patients. Good luck!"

He snorted in disgust and slammed the door. Simon heard a voice and answered the phone, then reported to me.

"Dr. Wegener is busy. His nurse says to call him later," Simon reported.

"What are we going to do?" Penny cried out.

I suctioned Rico's mouth and picked up the endoscope. Rico sputtered and looked dazed.

"I've cleaned his airway. I need to get back inside and get into the stomach. Raise up the head end of the bed as much as possible."

"He's pretty awake now, sir," Simon pointed out.

"I'm going to give him some more midazolam. Draw up another five milligrams."

"Another five? That won't be safe, Doctor," Penny protested.

"We don't have any options," I snapped. "And call CA. I need that magnet right now!"

Simon drew up the midazolam. He shook his head. I struggled to speak slowly and calmly.

"I know you don't approve. I've done this before. I think we still have a chance. Give Rico two milligrams IV now," I said.

Penny was alarmed. She grabbed my wrist.

"No! Don't do it! That's a big deal! Once you push it in, you can't get it out," she warned me.

I paused.

"You can push it in, but you can't pull it out!" Penny repeated.

"That's what the actress said to the bishop," Simon smirked, as he injected the sedative into Rico's vein.

Penny was appalled. She confronted Simon.

"How *dare* you? How dare you say that!" she stormed.

Simon shrugged sheepishly.

"Don't you *ever* talk like that in my presence again!" Penny seethed.

There was a knock at the door and Simon answered. He was given a plastic bag with a heavy object, the size of a coconut.

"CA retrieved a big magnet from a pump motor!" Simon said, brandishing a white bag.

"Wipe it and put it in a clean pillow case. Rico's getting sleepy," I said.

We watched and waited.

"He's still partially awake, sir," Simon said.

"Okay. Let's give him another milligram."

Penny shook her head silently and looked away. Simon obeyed.

"Pull back the corner of his face mask. I'm going in!" I said.

Rico jerked as the tube entered his throat and slid down to his stomach.

"He's not fighting you too much, Doctor," Penny noted.

"I realize that. It's not a good sign, it means that the medicine is building up."

"His breathing is pretty slow already."

"He might stop breathing. Keep that romazicon handy and get the crash cart in here and an eight and a half ET tube!"

I slid the tip of the scope past the oval ulcer where the battery had been stuck. The bleeding had slowed down. The stomach was a pool of glittering green and yellow fluid. Penny and Simon groaned loudly.

"How are you *ever* going to find that tiny little battery? There's all this muck everywhere!" Simon lamented.

"I'll try suctioning out as much as I can, maybe I can drain the stomach dry," I said.

I tried sucking the liquid out of Rico's stomach. The fluid level dropped at first, then the instrument shuddered and the fluid level remained steady.

"Crap!" Penny said. "Some stomach crap plugged up the scope. You want me to flush it, Doctor?"

"Yes, please."

Penny filled a sixty cc syringe with water and connected it to a side port on the instrument.

"Flush! Now!"

Penny thrust a syringeful of water through the scope and we watched anxiously. A granular yellowish-brown worm-shaped piece of debris shot out.

"Whoa! Bet that's what was blocking the scope!" Penny said.

"That's gross!" Simon recoiled.

"That's nothing," Penny chirped. "I'll show you gross. Green snot, blood in stools, pus from fistulas, *that's* gross. This is nothing!"

She flashed Simon a superior smile. Simon was not amused.

"I can't suction any more of this stuff, it's too thick," I said. I gazed at the debris in the stomach. Green bergs of partly digested bread and bacon floated to the surface.

I thrust the tip into the fluid and pumped in gas. It only produced thicker bubbles.

"Blowing in CO_2 isn't helping. I can't see a thing! Simon, put that magnet against his bellybutton! I'm going to shake up the stomach contents."

I moved the scope back and forth and sideways and tossed the contents around.

"Now turn him onto his back, but keep the magnet on his belly-button."

The three of us struggled to turn Rico from his side onto his back. An alarm screeched.

"Sir, his oxygen is eighty-three percent and falling!"

"He's had too much medicine! He's stopped breathing!" Penny cried.

"His oxygen's dropping and his breathing has slowed down, but not stopped. Draw up a vial of the antidote, romazicon."

"Should I inject it, sir?" Simon asked.

"Hold on! Once I give it, there's no going back. He'll wake right up and we won't be able to get that battery out," I said.

I watched the monitor. The oxygen level was eight-four percent.

"Wait a minute. I'm going to flush his stomach with water. The magnet may have pulled the battery out."

"Why are you waiting, Doctor? His oxygen is falling! It's now eighty-three percent! Get out of there!" Penny urged.

"Just give me a syringe of water. This is our chance!"

Penny handed me a sixty cc syringe of water. I injected it and washed the lining.

"There! There it is!" Penny cried out.

The disc battery, revealed itself, washed and shiny, stuck on the roof of the stomach directly underneath the magnet we had placed on his abdomen.

"Quick! Give me the Roth net!"

I slipped in the net and opened it up underneath the battery.

"Simon, remove the magnet now!"

The battery dropped easily into the open net. Penny closed the net and whooped.

"*Got it!* We *got* that sucker!"

"Sir, his oxygen's eighty-one percent," Simon warned.

"Give the romazicon. All of it, now!"

I pulled the scope out cautiously, wriggling the battery past the tight spots, then past the vocal cords and over the back of the tongue. I pulled the endoscope out completely. The net hung out of the tip, soggy and green, like a wet purse, with the battery inside. Simon held out a piece of gauze and Penny opened the net over it.

"It feels very warm," he said.

"It was inside the body," I reasoned.

"Sats now seventy-eight, dropping fast!" Simon warned.

I grasped Rico's jaw and pulled upwards.

"I'm going to keep the airway open. More oxygen! Go up to eight liters!"

I watched the monitor. The oxygen level started inching up.

Simon coughed.

"No, I mean, the battery is really warm. As in *abnormally* warm. I would call it hot," he said.

I touched the gauze and flinched.

"You're right! That's not body temperature. That battery's actually very hot!" I said.

We gazed at the small gauze pad with the battery inside. .

"Do you think it could explode?" Penny asked.

"I don't know. I don't think so. Simon, take it out and put it in an empty space in the parking lot and tell CA. Maybe he can watch it for us."

We rolled Rico back on his side.

"He breathes better on his side. When he lies flat on his back, his soft palate falls straight into his airway and obstructs him," I explained.

Rico woke up briefly, blinked, and went back to sleep. Five minutes passed slowly.

"His oxygen is up to ninety percent," Simon said.

Penny flushed and wiped the scope.

"Take that hot battery outside, Simon," she demanded. "*I'll* watch the patient."

Simon glanced at me. I nodded.

"The battery is hot. I've seen that happen, but I've never seen one explode," I said.

Simon picked it up gingerly and held it at arm's length. He had a curious look.

"Back in a jiffy," he said and shot out.

I watched Rico and scribbled my notes. Suddenly, there was a loud bang outside the ER, and a shower of pebbles hit the window. Penny jumped.

"Oh, my lands! Oh, sweet Jesus!" she cried.

I was astounded.

"The battery exploded! Doc, if you hadn't got it out in time, it would have exploded inside him and he would have died!" Penny wailed.

I was confused.

"If you hadn't got that battery out in time, it would have exploded in him!" Penny repeated.

Simon returned, his face flushed.

"CA dug a small hole. We threw the battery in it and poured water over it. Then it burst!" he said.

"The battery exploded! Sweet Jesus!" Penny shrieked. She was so upset that she shook. She sat down to steady herself.

"Can you imagine? Can you imagine if we hadn't got it out in time?" she shuddered. "What if it had exploded here in the ER?"

Simon looked as if he was about to say something, but checked himself. Penny held the side of the cart and pulled herself up.

"I'm going to get the endoscopy cart out of here and back upstairs to the OR and clean the scope and restock everything," she said, shakily. Simon gallantly held the door open for her.

I waited for a few minutes, then addressed Simon.

"I noticed that a large plastic bag went missing with you," I told Simon. Simon grinned.

"And the bang sounded like someone bursting a big plastic bag," I continued.

Simon shrugged.

"And there was a tiny delay before the dirt hit the window," I concluded. Simon nodded.

"You made up all those fireworks at the end of our little adventure, didn't you?"

"That's what the actress said to the bishop," Simon grinned.

CHAPTER 4
ONLY THE SPECIALIST, PLEASE

I entered the office through the back door. Karl stood by the coffee machine.

"Heard you got that dang battery out," Karl said.

"Uh huh," I tried to sound nonchalant.

"Hey, man, that was great! A little luck too, eh?"

"Very lucky. We managed to pull it out of the food with a big magnet."

"The one CA pulled out of a busted fan?"

"Yes."

Karl whistled.

"You're a specialist. You had two big cases today and you nailed them! You have skills. You are going to move to Abilene or Austin or some big city. You're not going to hang around Hotspur, no sir."

"I'm building up my practice here, Karl," I protested.

"What for? You're going to get up and leave anyway. So go ahead. You had three years on your contract, you're in the third year, you got your green cards. You did us good too, we all got what we wanted, right?"

"I'm comfortable here. I'm not planning to go anywhere," I said.

Karl shook his head in disbelief.

"I understand. That's the official version. Can't scare away the customers. Sit you down and get you some coffee."

He took a long sip and regarded his silver cylinder. Before I could avert my eyes, I read *Our Hero* in glittering letters. It bothered me. I refused to sit down.

"I have a patient waiting. Save me some coffee and a donut," I said.

"Have you not learnt anything? Have I not told you, never miss a meal for a patient?"

I shrugged.

"And anyway, she's gone to take a dump. Getting a fresh sample for you to study. So set you down and get you some java."

I sat down and pulled out a donut. Karl squinted at me.

"Maybe just half a donut," he suggested.

"What do you mean?"

"You're packing on the pounds. You're getting fat, dude."

I froze.

"Yeah. You're getting fat. You're a little guy. You need to lay off the free food. I see you eating the food the hospital sends you. Omelets and cheese sandwiches and stuff."

I put the donut down. My appetite evaporated.

"Seen yourself in a mirror lately?" Karl continued.

"Dr. Becker!" Tracy protested.

"Hush! Did I ask for your opinion?"

Tracy flushed.

"Did I? Did I ask for your opinion?"

Tracy blinked at her computer and remained silent.

"We got the Royal Physician to her imperial majesty the Queen of all England and someone who fancies himself as Dr. Sherlock Holmes, but he doesn't know he's packing on the pounds?"

"I got your point," I said.

"Good. Here's some coffee. Don't add sugar, buttercup."

He poured thick diesel-like fluid from a carafe into my cup. There was a whiff of green apples and lavender.

"Thanks," I muttered.

"You need a proper coffee container, like me. Hey, Trace!"

"Yes, sir."

"Order him one just like mine."

"Yes, sir."

"But not the same thing written on it. Mine says *Our Hero* and that's pretty corny, but whatever. His container should say something else."

Tracy scribbled a reminder.

"So what should they write on Dr. Mathur's coffee mug?" she asked.

Karl paused.

"Don't know. Let me think. Hey, Einstein! You think you're a great detective, right?"

"I look for clues and make guesses," I shrugged.

Karl snorted.

"You know why Gerta Gideon wants to see you and not me?"

"No."

"Because you're a specialist. I told her husband, Clyde, hey I reckon I know just as much as Sandy, I've been in practice longer, I can handle it. Guess what he said?"

I shrugged.

"He said, she only wants a specialist. Crazy, right?" Karl said.

I couldn't let that pass.

"I believe in specialists. You learn a lot more about a particular subject, there's a difference!" I steamed.

"Oh, so you're not just a lowly regular doc. You're a specialist! Oh, mama! A *specialist!*" Karl wagged his head and rolled his eyes. "Maybe your coffee mug should say *The Detective* or *The Specialist.*"

I sipped my coffee and gazed longingly at the donut.

"So when's Betty coming back from the hospital?" I asked.

Karl froze.

"How'd you know that?"

"A guess."

"Someone told you! Tracy! Did you tell him?" Karl accused.

"No sir! I did no such thing," Tracy snapped.

Karl spun around.

"Then who told you?" he asked.

"You did. You smell of her shampoo. Green apples and lavender."

"So what?"

"So you're using Betty's shampoo or soap or lotion. That means she hasn't been to Target to get your stuff. That only happens when she has to go to Amarillo for her mother."

"Lucky guess," Karl muttered and sat down. He opened a copy of *Guns And Ammo*.

"God has ways of keeping us humble," Tracy declared. Karl glared at her. Tracy smirked and returned to her work.

"So I got Betty's shampoo. Okay. So what? That's just a guess. Tell me something else, Sherlock. Surprise me."

I surveyed him. He glowered. He crossed his legs and sat back and slurped coffee.

"Tell me something and really surprise me and I'll get you a coffee container like mine."

I hesitated.

"I'll get it inscribed, too!" Karl added.

"You're practicing for a marathon," I said.

"I told you that," Karl scoffed.

"You're running on your driveway."

Karl shrugged.

"You got new running shoes."

Karl stopped drinking and stared at his coffee.

"And you're not drinking enough water," I concluded.

Karl slammed his hand on the table.

"So how did you know all that?" he demanded.

"You're wearing your running shoes right now. You would never do that unless you had a new pair and these were the old ones."

Karl looked at his shoes and shrugged. I drained my coffee and stood up.

"How'd you know about running on my driveway?"

"There's tar on your soles. You've got your main driveway newly paved but white caliche on the boundary roads."

"How'd you know about the water?"

"Everyone thinks they don't drink enough water. I just threw that in for the heck of it."

I walked out of the office.

Mrs. Gerta Gideon was in her mid-fifties. She was a plump lady, with short brown hair, bulging eyes and a receding chin. She sported matching silver earrings, necklace and bracelet and wore a snug pink dress, a white floppy hat, and matching white gloves. Her husband, Clyde, sat in the corner. He was considerably older, dressed simply in blue jeans and denim shirt, and gazed fixedly at an old white hat that he cradled in his lap. He sat silently. She held up her hand as I entered and spoke loudly.

"When people see me, they say, goodness, sugar, you're so much younger than your husband," she said. "And I say, you know what? It doesn't bother me."

I nodded and sat down.

"Good morning, Mr. and Mrs. Gideon. I'm Dr. Mathur," I said.

"I don't care about what people say. I don't care if Clyde, *dear* Clyde, is older than me. I love him and that's all that matters."

She turned around and blinked at Clyde. Clyde stared at his hat. She turned back to me.

"Dr. Mathur, I need your help desperately," she whispered.

"I'm here to help."

"*Desperately!*"

I nodded sympathetically.

"I need your help so badly I could cry!"

"What's the problem, exactly?" I asked.

Mrs. Gideon took a deep breath.

"You're a specialist, right?" she asked.

"Yes."

"I heard you trained in Houston and London and studied for years and saw thousands of patients."

"Yes, ma'am, that's true."

"Baylor in Houston and some Royal something in London?"

"I've been in medicine a long time, yes."

"You've written stuff, the local paper said. Medical stuff. Research. Is that true?"

"Yes."

"*Hundreds* of things?"

"No. Actually, I have about ten publications."

Mrs. Gideon stiffened.

"Just ten?"

"They were in good journals, but yes, only ten publications."

"In journals that were read by *thousands* of doctors?"

"Well, some of the journals might have been read by a few hundred, maybe even a thousand. But these are specialty journals, so they don't have a lot of readers."

Mrs. Gideon scowled.

"The *Hotspur Herald* is read by over three thousand people," she sniffed.

"I realize that."

"Twice weekly, mind you."

I nodded.

"So what, exactly, is the problem?" I asked, attempting to focus.

Mrs. Gideon sat back and gazed at me with frank disappointment.

"I thought that you were a famous specialist from Houston, who had done great work, and whose work had been praised by thousands of other specialists," she lamented. "I was wrong. Even our local paper has more readers."

"But I am a specialist," I assured her.

"Where, exactly, did you study?" she asked, bluntly.

"Baylor and M.D. Anderson, and the University of Texas."

She softened.

"M.D. Anderson?" she murmured.

"Yes. I did my research there."

She rested her head on one shoulder, then the other. She straightened up and turned around.

"What do you think, Clyde?"

Clyde kept staring at his hat.

"Clyde!"

Clyde shrugged, but didn't look up.

"Oh, alright. I guess if you went to Baylor and M.D. Anderson and all, and you're a specialist, I guess I gotta trust you."

I held my breath. She leaned forwards to deliver the revelation. I leaned in, cautiously.

"It's about my turds," she whispered.

I was surprised. I straightened up.

"My turds are all messed up," she said.

"What do you mean?"

"Sometimes they're mushy and nice, like soft-serve ice cream, nice color like sienna brown in a sixty-four box of crayons. But sometimes they're green and slimy and even frothy like doggy throw-up."

I looked at her. I didn't know what to say. Mrs. Gideon pressed on.

"Sometimes they're small and hard, like goat turds, and sometimes they come out round and flat like sand dollars, sometimes round and shiny as marbles. I had one that looked like a smiley-face, one like two kids holding hands, and the other day I did a real curly one like a shrimp with little legs and all! Today, I had one like a boomerang with a couple of pointy bits sticking out. Looked like it was giving me thumbs up. Then one looked like a billy club and another like a snake with a rattle!"

Clyde blinked as he gripped his wide-brimmed hat. He seemed to be suppressing some emotion.

"Sometimes they're big. Had one that shot out like a cannonball, nearly busted the commode. The next day it was like soft serve ice-cream again, and then, a real hard one with ridges, looked like a salt shaker."

Mrs. Gideon stared at me, her eyes widening as she spoke. Clyde blinked furiously and shuddered. The hat wobbled and he steadied it.

"One yesterday had two parts, big and little, like two jelly beans joined by a toothpick. Another, so much like a scorpion, I nearly called Clyde in to check and see."

"Why didn't you?" I asked.

"Because in a minute I covered it with soft-serve. I waited to see if it would come back up, and when it didn't I figured I killed it."

I looked at her and wondered whether she was joking. She was not. Her eyes widened and her voice rose with agitation.

Mrs. Gideon pursed her lips and paused and gazed at me to see if I could be trusted. I remained impassive.

"Had some with round hard bits *and* soft serve, looked like an old man's face, and then I did two little bitty things that bounced right off it like bullets," Mrs. Gideon complained.

I didn't know what to say.

"Then I passed a baby duck and another looked like an oyster on the half-shell," she continued.

Clyde shook with suppressed laughter. To my horror, I heard Karl snickering outside.

"Sometimes, the soft serve even has hard bits deep inside," Mrs. Gideon continued. "Last week, I passed a couple hard stools that looked like a pair of boots, and then the strangest thing, Doctor!"

"What?" I asked.

"Then I passed the leprechaun that was wearing the boots!"

Karl roared outside. I closed my eyes for a minute. Karl had heard everything. Mrs. Gideon paused dramatically.

"It was a leprechaun," she insisted. "It had a hat and head and belly and arms but no legs."

"No legs?"

"They came out with the boots, I reckon."

I nodded. Clyde snickered.

"Is there something wrong?" she inquired.

"Nothing. Nothing at all," I gulped. "Where were we?"

"I was talking about the leprechaun," Mrs. Gideon said.

I blinked and nodded.

"Very serious," Mrs. Gideon observed. "A parasite, don't you think?"

I still didn't know what to say. I just sat and stared. Mrs. Gideon arched back and pinched her lips to deliver the greatest surprise of all.

"But this morning my turd was a *python!* One end was pointy and the other end had a bunch of little round hard turds like a rattler. All curled up like a snake!"

Clyde shook with suppressed laughter. I heard Karl sniggering outside. Mrs. Gideon turned back to chastise Clyde.

"Clyde! Clyde! Darling!" she appealed.

Clyde controlled himself and gripped his hat so tightly he mangled the brim. Mrs. Gideon threw her hands up.

"The man's a *specialist,*" Mrs. Gideon explained. "He *needs* to hear this!"

Clyde had a final tremor, then steadied himself under his wife's unrelenting glare.

"This man *needs* to hear all this. He's a *specialist,*" she repeated, gravely.

She pointed to me, while still glaring at him.

"He's a specialist, a *specialist in shit,*" she announced.

My mouth fell open. Mrs. Gideon turned back to me for affirmation.

"Right? You're a specialist, right, a specialist in shit?" she asked.

I looked at her, astonished. I heard Karl laughing outside. I knew he had heard everything.

But Mrs. Gideon gazed back at me, wide-eyed, with the awe of an entomologist studying a rare dung beetle.

"You've been to London and you're some kind of Royal specialist," she went on. "You even know about English turds?"

"I'm a gastroenterologist," I explained, weakly parsing reality.

Mrs. Gideon nodded and turned back to Clyde in triumph.

"Hah! See? I was right. He studied in London and everywhere, so he's a *world specialist* in shit," she declared.

Clyde remained motionless but I heard Karl guffawing outside.

I swallowed.

"I've taken pictures of everything," Mrs. Gideon announced.

I held up my hand.

"That's fine. You've been very helpful already. Your explanations have been so helpful."

"You don't want to see my album?"

"Not necessary. I commend your diligence. I have some recommendations about your diet," I said. "I'm going to talk to you about a high fiber diet."

"Will that fix my turds?" she demanded.

"Yes."

Mrs. Gideon sat back and placed her hands on her knees and regarded me with satisfaction.

"See, Clyde? I was right! You got a problem with shit, you gotta come to the shit specialist!" she said, triumphantly.

I kept a low profile the rest of the day. As I sneaked out of the clinic that evening, Karl spotted me.

"God has ways of keeping us modest, right?" he said, with a big grin.

I didn't answer.

I hoped that was the last of it, but it wasn't.

Days later, a small box arrived for me. I opened it in my office. It was a stainless steel coffee container, a gift from Karl, with an inscription that made me wince: *Shit Specialist*.

It still sits on my desk, years and years later. It keeps my coffee warm and my life unpretentious.

CHAPTER 5
IT'S COMPLICATED

As I stepped into the hospital parking lot, I saw a one-armed man in a green paisley shirt and denim overalls reclining against the oxygen cylinder and smoking. He saw me and stood up. His empty sleeve was folded up and pinned close at the shoulder. The man turned away, puffing hurriedly. He waved as I walked past him and entered the building. I had a premonition: this day would be different.

I went upstairs to the second floor. Across from the clinic, there was a swinging door that opened into a small hallway next to the Operating Room. We used it to prepare patients for procedures and to recover them afterwards. I had a patient scheduled for a colonoscopy. The OR nurse, Penny, had changed our patient into a hospital gown and had started an IV. She had our patient lying down in bed, covered with warm blankets. She beamed as I entered.

"There you are! Dr. Mathur, this is Mrs. Frankie Washington. She's here for a colonoscopy," Penny said.

Mrs. Washington was a thin, round-faced African-American lady with a halo of crisp white hair. She had a veneer of make-up and smelled of soap. She smiled broadly and nodded.

"Thank you for getting her ready. Good morning, Mrs. Washington."

"Good morning!"

"How are you this morning?"

"Still hurting, Doc."

"Did the pain get worse with the prep?"

"Yes, it did. Even bled a little."

I reviewed the chart.

"You're seventy-two years old, married, live here in Hotspur, and you're a retired business owner. You take prednisone five milligrams daily and lisinopril ten milligrams daily. Allergic to sulfa drugs. You've had a hysterectomy but no other surgery. Correct so far?"

"Yes. After that hysterectomy, I swore I would never ever have another surgery."

"Why are you taking prednisone?"

"I have lupus."

"How long have you been on prednisone?"

"Couple three years at least."

"Did you take a booster dose of prednisone today?"

"No. Should I?"

"Yes. Prednisone is a steroid. Your body is supposed to make its own steroids all the time. When you take prednisone by mouth daily, your body stops making steroids because you're supplying them. The problem is that when you undergo some stress, like an operation or a procedure, you need a boost of steroids but your body has already switched off production."

"So I need to take some extra prednisone before an operation or procedure?"

"Exactly. It's safer if I give you some steroids by vein right now, so we can start our test."

Mrs. Washington smiled.

"Sure. Go right ahead, Doctor."

I turned to Penny.

"Solu-Medrol forty milligrams IV now, please," I ordered. Penny nodded and disappeared. I turned back to Mrs. Washington.

"Let me examine you."

I listened to her heart and lungs and palpated her abdomen. She winced when I pressed on the lower part of her abdomen. I noticed that she had a long transverse scar in the lower part of the abdomen, below her umbilicus, and several smaller scars on either side.

"Did you have complications after your hysterectomy?" I asked.

"I sure did! I was in the hospital for thirty-nine days after the surgery.

Thirty-nine days! I thought I was never going to get out of there! I had an infection and they had to open me up twice to clean it all up. Had drains sticking out of me."

"Is that why you said you would never have another operation?"

"Yes. It was terrible."

I thought about it. Mrs. Washington looked at me.

"Is that going to be a problem, Doc?" she asked.

"It might. It could mean that you have scar tissue there and that could cause your intestines to get all tangled up."

"Could it be causing my pain?"

"It's possible. But it increases the risk of the procedure. If the intestine is twisted up then the instrument might scratch it and hurt it."

"I understand."

"The worst thing that could happen is a tear, a perforation, where the instrument pokes a hole in the intestine."

Mrs. Washington was alarmed.

"What? Poke a hole in the intestine?"

"It's rare, but it could happen."

She covered her mouth with her hand and shook her head. The door opened and the one-armed man entered. He was tall, white, and had meat chop sideburns. He stretched out his left and we shook.

"B.B. Washington, proud to meet you. I reckoned it was you in the parking lot. What kind of car you drive?"

"It's a Toyota Corolla."

"One of them fancy little imports. Doc, you got to get you a truck. That little bitty thing don't cut it here."

His wife grabbed his belt.

"Honey, the Doc just told me he might punch a hole in my intestine!"

BB was incredulous.

"What do you mean, Doc?" he asked.

"Your wife had lots of problems after her hysterectomy and there could be scar tissue."

"But that was years and years ago!"

"Yes, but the scar tissue could still be there. It could have twisted up the intestines and that might be what's hurting her."

"So what should we do? Go for surgery?" he asked.

"No, no surgeon would operate without being sure of the diagnosis. We would need to check the intestine and see what's going on. We could send her to Abilene for an x-ray test called a barium enema."

Mrs. Washington let out a roar of protest.

"Oh, no! Oh, no! I'm never doing that again! They tried that once, no sir, never again! They stuck that big old plastic hose up my rear end and shot that white chalky stuff into me! It was awful!"

"But it would be safer than the colonoscopy," I argued.

"I'm not doing the enema test," Mrs. Washington declared, flatly.

"She ain't doing it," B.B. concurred.

We looked at each other.

"Doc, go ahead. Do the colon scope," Mrs. Washington said.

"Well, hold on, Mama," B.B. said. "Wait a cotton-picking minute. What if there's a tear? Then what?"

"Then we would have to go to Abilene and have a surgeon open her up and stitch the tear closed."

The Washingtons looked at each other.

"You said you never wanted to have another operation," I reminded her.

Mrs. Washington looked at me squarely.

"I trust you. You're not going to do anything wrong. You have experience, I'm going to say a prayer, all will be well."

"Do you want to discuss it with BB? I can come back in a few minutes," I offered.

"No. I heard you did a couple real difficult cases here and you did great. I believe in you, Doctor. I think the Lord wants me to go ahead," Mrs. Washington said.

BB held up his hand.

"How much experience do you have in these kinda procedures, Doc?" he asked.

Before I could answer, the door was flung open and Karl strode in.

"Hey man! You done?" he asked.

"No. I haven't even started."

"Why not? How long does it take a Royal Specialist from London to do a darn colonoscopy?"

"I was explaining the risks of the procedure."

"You're a specialist, you've done a bunch of these, right?"

"Yes, I have."

"How many, ace?"

"At least a thousand. Maybe two thousand."

"Dang! That's a bunch!" Karl said. He looked at the Washingtons and gave a thumbs-up. BB looked at his wife.

"This guy's great! I saw him work on two real difficult cases Monday and he fixed 'em both. He's good!" Karl declared.

The Washingtons smiled nervously.

"Dang good for a foreigner!" Karl added, "Heck, I'd let Sandy operate on my family, he's *that* good!"

I felt a surge of gratitude. The Washingtons nodded, reassured.

"But there could still be complications," I added.

Karl was irritated.

"What did I tell you last time? You got to be confident, man! You got experience, you got knowledge, but you *got* to get confidence. Go for it!"

Karl turned around and returned to the door. He stopped and pointed at me.

"Almost forgot what I came for. We got a drug rep from Dallas, brought us a bunch of bagels and cream cheese and smoked salmon. We just made us fresh coffee. He wants to do a presentation, wants you to be there. Hurry up and get your royal backside over to my office!"

I turned to the Washingtons.

"There are risks of this procedure including tearing the lining, bleeding, infections, and drug reactions, and the risks could be very bad, even fatal. That means, you could die from them," I warned.

"I understand the risks, Doctor. I'll sign the consent form," Mrs. Washington said.

"You understand and accept the risks?" I persisted. "I won't be upset if you cancel."

The Washingtons had made up their minds.

"Go ahead, Doc. Mama wants you to do it. Just be careful. We'll be praying for you," B.B. said. He shook my shoulder warmly. He kissed his wife on the forehead, held her hand and said a short prayer, and left the room.

"Okay, then!" Penny cried, and tucked the loose blankets and covers under the mattress. She secured the IV pole to the side and we wheeled the bed into the Operating Room.

The OR was a windowless chamber, fourteen by eighteen feet, with white tiled floors and walls. One long side had slender wooden cabinets and a narrow ledge. A large operating room lamp had been flipped to illuminate the ceiling. The endoscopy cart, with its small monitor, was parked next to the cabinets and the patient was wheeled around it. We connected her to oxygen and monitors.

"Let me show you the endoscope," I said.

I held up the endoscope, a long thin black tube.

"It looks like a snake," Mrs. Washington declared.

"That it does," Penny agreed. "Now put your head down on the pillow, darling, and relax. The doctor is going to give you a little medicine and make you go to sleep."

We turned our patient gently onto her left side.

"I'm giving you some medicine in your vein right now. It may burn a little as it goes in," I warned.

"That hurts!" Mrs. Washington cried. "It burns like fire!"

"It will get better."

Mrs. Washington groaned and shifted.

"I'm going to wait a few minutes, then maybe give you a little more."

"How much have you given, Doc?" Penny asked.

"She's had two point five of midazolam and twenty-five of meperidine."

"She looks pretty drowsy," Penny said.

We waited a few minutes. Mrs. Washington was still restless.

"I'm giving her another one point five of midazolam," I announced. Penny recorded it.

We watched the monitor. The patient's heart rate settled down and her oxygen saturation remained steady. Her breathing slowed down and became quiet and regular.

"I think she's asleep now," Penny said, and turned the lights out.

I checked the endoscope by placing the tip in a small container of water and suctioning water in and bubbling air out of the instrument. I did a quick rectal exam. The anus was normal and the rectal vault was empty.

"I'm placing the tip of the scope in the rectum now. I can see that the cleanout is good, I can see the lining clearly. But the next part of the colon is pretty twisted up."

I advanced the tip towards the top of the rectum and tried to enter the sigmoid colon.

"This area is pretty tight. I'm twisting the scope and applying a little pressure, but I'm not getting anywhere," I said.

"What should we do?"

"Let's roll her onto her back. That should help."

We rolled Mrs. Washington onto her back. Suddenly, the angle changed and I could see the way forward.

"Good. I can see the lumen, so I'm going to advance."

I pushed forwards, but met resistance again.

"This is frustrating. The sigmoid colon is very tight. I'm having a hard time getting through."

"Should we re-position her?"

"No, I don't think it would help. Give me an upper endoscope."

"You mean, the endoscope we use for the stomach?"

"Yes. It's much thinner so it should be better for this narrow area."

"Why didn't you start with it?" Penny asked as she changed the instruments.

"The upper scope is much shorter than the colonoscope, so we may not be able to get to the very end of the colon. But we first need to get through this narrow area to make any progress at all."

The door was flung open and Dr. Becker strode in.

"Einstein! You done?" he asked.

"No. Barely started."

"What's the matter? The specialist can't get it done?" he mocked.

"The sigmoid colon is very tight. I'm changing scopes."

"Man, we are waiting on you. This drug rep, he's something else. He's got all this great food, wants to do this presentation, but won't start till you get there."

"Let me finish, I'll be right there."

"Hurry up! That drug rep's got an attitude and he's pissing me off."

I slipped the tip of the smaller endoscope into the rectum and it easily entered the sigmoid colon.

"Just hurry up!" Karl repeated.

I pushed ahead and again stopped.

"What's the matter, ace?"

"There's some resistance. I don't know if I should push ahead a little or pull back."

Karl snorted.

"You're the specialist. You got the Royal kiss of approval from her majesty, right? So you just do whatever the heck you want, Einstein. Just hurry up!"

I pushed forwards gently. More resistance. I pulled back and tried another angle. No better.

"Let's get her back on her side."

We moved her back onto her side.

"I'm going to push a tiny bit harder," I said.

Suddenly, there was a new vista. I saw a large cavity, lined with yellow buntings of fat, soft grey tubes of intestine, and a snatch of brown liver in the distance. My mouth turned to sand and I felt faint. I couldn't breathe.

"What in tarnation is *that*?" Karl wondered.

I had frozen completely in horror. I couldn't breathe or speak.

"What the heck is *that*?" Karl repeated. "Where the heck are you?"

I hastily pulled the scope out.

"I was in the peritoneal cavity," I admitted.

"What?" Karl blared. "*What*? The peritoneal cavity?"

"What does that mean, Doc?" Penny asked.

"It means that I perforated the colon."

There was a shocked silence.

"You mean you, like, tore through the colon?" Penny asked, incredulously.

"Yes," I croaked, still dazed.

"Are you sure?"

"Yes," I said. I revisited the image seared in my brain. The glistening cavity, the smooth greyish-green intestines, the rubbery maroon liver. There was no question.

"Hoo-wee," Karl declared. "Man, you really screwed the pooch!"

"Dr. Becker!" Penny complained.

"What? He screwed up royally. He just perforated the dang colon!"

Karl did not sound devastated. On the contrary, his voice had a hint of jubilation.

"No bagels and cream cheese for you, eh?" he said.

"Her vital signs are stable, but I need to get her to a surgeon right away," I croaked.

"Let me call old Rusty Morgan," Karl offered. "We went to medical school together. He's a general surgeon in Abilene, at Abilene Memorial."

I nodded. I was still in shock.

"You need to go talk to her old man," Karl advised.

"Yes."

"He's that one-armed guy, right?"

"Yes."

"Heard he's got a vicious temper!"

I swallowed.

"Better stand six feet back when you tell him what you've done!"

I didn't know what to say.

"Better break it gently, ace. Maybe take Penny with you, in case he starts swinging."

"Dr. Becker! He's not like that!" Penny protested.

"Was the old man packing heat?" Karl went on, happily.

"What do you mean?"

"What do I mean, Einstein? I mean, was the old man armed? Is he carrying a gun? He shouldn't be, not inside the hospital, it's against rules. But just be sure he isn't. Wouldn't want him to start shooting at you."

I was turning to jelly. Karl whipped out a large cell phone and punched in a number.

"Dr. Mathur, don't worry! BB's not going to hit you or shoot you!" Penny reassured me.

"Yeah? Well, tell that to Sandy's wife, at the funeral, okay?"

"You're just saying all that to scare Dr. Mathur."

"Heck, I'm just trying to save Sandy's ass. Look, I'm on hold for Naunton Morgan, so get you out there and talk to the husband, and I'll keep an eye on your patient."

Penny hesitated.

"Both of you better go! Hurry!"

Penny looked at Karl in confusion.

"What? You don't want to go? You worried he might hit you or shoot you instead?" Karl sniggered.

Penny marched to the door.

"Let's go, Doc!" she said.

"Hey, be sure to duck! Make sure he doesn't get your head or chest," Karl drawled as we left. We removed our masks and gloves and stepped out.

"Don't let him get a head shot," Karl called out behind us.

We found BB in the waiting area just outside the ER. He struggled to his feet and stood up stiffly.

"How'd it go, Doc?" he asked.

I stared him in the face.

"It didn't go well. I have bad news. I had just started the test and I wasn't able to get through the colon with the regular instrument. I changed to a smaller instrument, but it didn't work. I tore the lining and made a hole in the colon."

BB was shocked. He held on to the top of a chair for support.

"The colon was very twisted. I tried to move her from side to side, changed the position, and changed to a smaller instrument. But when I gave a little pressure, the tip burst through the colon."

BB gaped at me in panic.

"So what we gonna do now?" BB asked.

"We need to take her to Abilene to see a surgeon so he can repair the hole, put a few stitches in it and fix it."

"You know, she said no more operations, Doc," BB pointed out.

"Yes. But this is an emergency. She has to have this."

"Can we fix it without surgery?"

"No. She absolutely has to have surgery."

BB nodded.

"Then let's do it. Let's get her to Abilene."

I nodded.

"Can I ride in the ambulance with her?" BB asked.

"Yes. In fact, I'm going to be with her too, in the ambulance," I said.

"Is she bad?"

"No, I just want to be there and get her to the surgeon safely."

BB suddenly reached into his back pocket. I stiffened.

"Whoa!" Penny yelped.

BB pulled out a large red handkerchief and blew his nose.

"Dang allergies!" he complained.

We settled Mrs. Washington into a stretcher. She was groggy.

"What happened?" she mumbled.

"We're taking you to Abilene," Penny said, cheerfully.

"Abilene! Why?"

"Because you need to see a surgeon. Hold on, I'm going to strap you in."

I examined Mrs. Washington again. She had no bowel sounds at all.

"Why do I need to see a surgeon?"

"Because Dr. Mathur made a little hole in your intestine," Penny answered, calmly.

"Oh," Mrs. Washington said, sleepily. "Okay."

"Are you hurting, Mrs. Washington?" I asked.

"No, I'm not."

"You might start hurting pretty soon as the medicine wears off. We're getting an ambulance in a few minutes. I'm coming with you to Abilene. Dr. Becker called his friend Dr. Morgan, who is a surgeon, and he will be waiting for us at the ER."

"How bad is it?"

"It's not too bad right now, but you might start hurting pretty soon. Don't worry, I'll be with you. Let me get my white coat and I'll be back."

Penny caught my hand as I left.

"Take a breather. She's okay, she's stable, and the ambulance will be here in ten minutes. They were out in the country and they're headed right back."

"Okay, thanks."

"Get yourself a coffee."

I shook my head and shot out. Eating was the last thing on my mind.

"Hey, there's our specialist!" Karl cried out, as I tore through the office.

A tall man of massive proportions stood up. He had the physique of a bull; his neck was the size of a tree trunk and he grabbed my hand with the strength that would have throttled a wolf. He wore a dark suit that resisted closure and a stringy tie that hung like a leash.

"Cassius P. Sanders, pleased to meet you!" he boomed.

I tried to wrench my hand loose.

"I'm sorry, I have to go. I can't come to your presentation."

"How about a bagel and some salmon and a quick cup of coffee?" he offered, not letting go of my hand.

"I just want to get my white coat and go," I said.

Karl shook his head in mock sorrow.

"One day you're the peacock, next day you're the feather duster," he smirked.

Cassius stared at me with curiosity. Karl waved towards the food.

"Have a cup of coffee, ace! The ambulance isn't here yet. What are you going to do, play dominoes with BB?" he chuckled.

Cassius pulled me over to a table near the coffee machine and offered a bagel slathered with cream cheese. A chair appeared behind me.

"Sit you down, Einstein," Karl said.

I sat down. I took a few deep breaths and bit into the bagel.

"I want to talk to you doctors about our new, wonderful arthritis medicine," Cassius said, grandly. "A totally new advance in the field! Very exciting!"

Tracy brought me a cup of coffee. Karl nodded, approvingly.

"How do you like your coffee, Dr. Becker?" Cassius asked.

"Hot and black, just like I like my women," Karl answered.

He grinned as Cassius stood with his mouth open for a few seconds.

"Give us the pitch," Karl ordered.

Cassius recovered and began.

"Our new medicine, Arthur-Right-Is, has an anti-inflammatory for the inflammation and a pain control medicine for the pain, and vitamin D for the bones."

Karl snorted. He took a giant bite of a bagel.

"So your exciting new medicine is actually three old medicines," he said, dismissively.

"It's the brilliant combination, that's what makes the difference! You see, we've covered all the parts of arthritis. And the anti-inflammatory part is really new!"

"So what? It's just like ibuprofen and all the others."

"No, it's not. It's much better. It's specially made so it does not harm the stomach, that's why I was so excited for Dr. Mathur to use it. It only works on the joints and it does not hurt the stomach. No stomach ulcers!"

"Big deal," Karl grunted.

"Dr. Mathur, you can appreciate this. I can understand if a family practice guy can't appreciate it, but surely *you* can. Surely you know that anti-inflammatory medicines like ibuprofen can cause stomach ulcers."

"Everyone knows that!" I said, irritated.

"Even if others don't know or care, I hope *you* know and care."

"I just said, yes, I do know."

Cassius gazed at Karl and me with concern.

"I realize that when you live out here, so far away from the real world, you do get kind of disconnected," Cassius said.

Karl and I stared at each other.

"I understand if you guys are a little rusty. Maybe you don't really know much about recent advances."

Karl glared at him.

"You guys went to medical school a long, long time ago, so it's natural you would be out of touch," Cassius went on.

Karl slammed his hand on the table.

"You are peddling a selective COX-2 inhibitor that has been juiced up with old acetaminophen and plain vitamin D, and you tell us it's something new and exciting. *You're* the one who's out of touch, my man!"

Cassius shrugged.

"Don't get heated up. Just sit back and learn something today. Give your arthritis patients this nice new medicine and they will stop coming back. You won't have to see them again and again. We even made the name easy for country docs like you. Arthur-Right-Is!"

"We're not hick doctors!" Karl growled. "We're board certified and Sandy's even certified by the Royal Queen of England. She personally knighted him and then kicked his brown butt all the way to Texas! We take care of this little town pretty damn well!"

Cassius shrugged.

"Who would live here, in this little town, away from everything? Who would practice here? You all must be pretty desperate to live here, hiding your secrets, intermarrying and all, I guess. None of my business. I just thought I would be your teacher, you know, bring a little knowledge into this dark corner of Texas."

Cassius looked so sincere that Karl and I were astonished.

"Just upgrade you," Cassius added. "I'm feeling charitable. I want to help."

Karl stood up abruptly and stopped. He must have considered Cassius' neck and chest and arms and decided not to punch him. He clenched his fists and stomped to the window instead.

"Your ambulance just showed up, Sandy. You better go. I'll clean up with God's Gift from Dallas here."

CHAPTER 6

THE ROAD TO ABILENE

We rolled Mrs. Washington up to the ambulance doors. She was strapped tightly to the stretcher and the IV fluids hung from a pole. The stretcher wheels folded and she slid straight inside. The stretcher was secured to the floor in six places. There were two slim metal benches on either side. I sat on her right side along with the paramedic, Derek. Her husband, BB, sat on her other side. He leaned forwards and squeezed her wrist with his hand. I checked her IV and her monitors and the leads and examined her again. She smiled weakly.

"Don't look so worried, Doc, I'm going to be just fine," she reassured me.

"I'm just checking everything," I said.

"You look so worried! Don't be so worried," Mrs. Washington said.

"God doesn't make mistakes, Doc," BB said, calmly.

I looked at him.

"God doesn't make mistakes, Doc. I believe that," he reiterated.

"I think I did, though," I said.

"God was with you, and God moves in strange and wondrous ways, His miracles to perform," BB said. Derek nodded.

The driver looked back and shouted.

"We're ready! Y'all ready?"

Derek gave him thumbs up. The ambulance siren howled and the vehicle shuddered and lurched forward. We swerved past the oxygen tanks, bounced over the parking lot and landed heavily on College Street. The siren grew louder and sharper as we accelerated towards the highway. The ambulance rattled and shook a lot more than I expected.

"Never been in an ambulance before, Doc?" Derek asked.

"Not in Texas. I've been in one in London, and in Bahrain, and they were much smaller. This is like being shaken inside a big metal can."

"Yeah, it's big. We got oxygen, we got meds, we got IV fluids and all kinds of bandages and supplies, back braces and such, you name it."

The heart monitor started beeping loudly.

"Her heart rate is shooting up, Doc!" Derek yelped.

"Mrs. Washington, your heart rate is going up. Are you hurting?" I asked.

"No."

"Now, Mama!" BB said, sternly.

"No, I'm not hurting," Mrs. Washington said, stoically.

"Your heart rate is a hundred and thirty. That's high. It may be due to pain or loss of fluid."

"I'm not hurting," Mrs. Washington repeated.

"Mama! You just told me that you were hurting pretty bad in the hospital," BB said.

"Not hurting," Mrs. Washington insisted, and looked away.

"Doc, she just told me that she was hurting pretty bad," BB revealed.

"Mrs. Washington, you may be leaking fluid out of your intestine. I'm going to speed up your fluids. I'm increasing your fluids to four hundred cc an hour," I said. I reached out and adjusted the flow rate.

Derek leaned forward.

"Isn't that a lot of fluid? She won't get fluid overloaded?" he asked.

"It sounds like a lot, I know. But she was getting two hundred cc an hour and I'm giving her another two hundred. We are going to be in Abilene in about fifty minutes so she won't get more than two hundred extra cc."

"Still sounds like a lot, Doc."

I nodded. Derek persisted.

"My grandma, they thought she had double pneumonia, gave her a bunch of fluids and she nearly died! Almost killed her! She had heart failure, they gave her too much doggone fluid, Doc, nearly killed her!"

"But Mrs. Washington does not have congestive failure. Also I'm not giving her that much extra."

"But you increased it from two hundred to four hundred cc, Doc!"

"Do you know how many cc there are in a small coffee cup?"

"Nope. Not sure. "

"About one hundred and twenty cc. So I'm giving her an extra cup and a half of coffee over fifty minutes."

"That doesn't sound too much, then," Derek nodded, relieved.

We watched the monitor and scrutinized our patient. Her heart rate remained high.

"Doc, her heart rate is still high. Are you sure about the fluids?" Derek asked again.

"Mrs. Washington, do you have any heart disease like congestive heart failure or heart attacks?"

"No, and I want you to call me Frankie."

I watched the monitor. I was worried. I listened to her heart and lungs and examined her abdomen. "Your heart sounds good and your lungs are clear. I don't feel your abdomen swelling up with fluid leaking out."

"If the abdomen isn't swelling up then where's the fluid going?" Derek asked. "You said the lungs are clear so there's no fluid there. Then where's the fluid going?"

"The fluid is leaking into the abdomen. It's just not enough to make her belly bulge."

Derek looked unconvinced.

"She's lying on her back and the fluid is pooling on both sides of her spine. We call that space the para-vertebral gutters," I explained.

BB looked at me, alarmed.

"Doc, are you sure? Does Frankie need more fluids? You sure about this?" he asked.

"Based on my experience, that's the right diagnosis. But we're in an ambulance so I can't really confirm it by doing an X-ray or CT scan. I have to go with my best guess."

BB looked at me.

"Let's say you're right, Doc. You're giving her fluids like you think she needs. But her heart rate is still very high. How come she's not getting better?"

I hesitated.

"Maybe I haven't given her enough fluids," I said.

"If you're right, her heart rate should have slowed down," Derek pointed out.

"I agree. Her heart rate should have settled down as I replaced the fluids but it hasn't gone down. I may need to give more."

"But if she's got some kind of heart problem like my grandma, you'll make it worse with more fluids!" Derek said.

I mentally reviewed Frankie's course. I felt my diagnosis was correct but there's always that element of doubt in medicine. I remembered Karl Becker's advice about projecting confidence.

I straightened up and changed my tone.

"I've thought about it and I'm sure," I said, with authority. I leaned forward and turned the IV valve wide open. Saline poured down like a stream.

"Whoa! Doc! You're giving her *lots* of fluids!" Derek protested.

I waved him down. We waited anxiously. Within minutes, the heart rate slowed down. I breathed again.

"Frankie, your vital signs are much better. I can give you a little morphine now," I said. "I think you're hurting. You wince every time we hit a bump, and that means the lining of the abdomen has become irritated."

"I don't want any dope."

"Dope? It's not dope, it's a painkiller for the serious damage that you have. The fluid leaking out of your intestine is burning up the lining of the abdominal cavity. You need morphine for pain control."

"It's dope and I don't want any part of it."

BB shook his head.

"It's okay, Mama. It's dope, but you're not taking it for fun. Go ahead and take it."

"No. I'm not hurting."

"I can see your eyes pinching from the pain. Everytime we hit a bump, it throws you and you hurt! I can see it in your eyes," BB said.

"No dope, BB. I'm okay."

BB shook his head and turned to me.

"Doc, I used to do drugs. That's why she won't take morphine. I used to shoot up my left arm and got gangrene in it. But that's not what got it cut off, no sir."

"Mrs. Washington, I think you need a little dose of morphine. You'll be more comfortable," I urged.

"No, Doctor. No morphine."

We stared at her. She clenched her eyes and gritted her teeth. Her face turned red and she gasped as we hit potholes.

Derek turned to BB.

"So how'd you lose the arm?" Derek asked.

BB laughed.

"It was the craziest thing. I was water-skiing. I was really good at it, you know. We were on Hord's Creek Lake, and I was with my girlfriend at that time. I wrapped the cord around my left hand and forearm and waved to my buddy who was driving the boat. Well, that sucker just took off like a son of a gun! Plumb ripped my whole arm out!"

Derek whistled.

"Ripped your arm out? Man, that must have been painful!" he said.

"You know, I don't remember much after that. I remember being pulled out of the water and someone in the hospital asking me my name but the rest, well, that's just a blur. I ended up with phantom pains in my limb that was gone. So I started on serious pain meds."

"How'd you meet your wife?" Derek asked.

"She was my nurse," BB grinned. "Black nurse looking after a white boy.

She changed my life forever."

Frankie Washington groaned.

"Well, now as I've begun the story I might as well tell you. When I went to the hospital with my arm gone I was already in trouble with the police."

"What kind of trouble?" Derek asked.

"Well, petty theft, brawling, some bar fights, you know. Just a stupid kid."

"But you straightened out," Derek pointed out.

"You know, that's the strange thing. See, when I was a little kid, my mother walked out on us. My dad, he went and remarried, and his second wife was real mean. I hated coming home so I hung out with my friends after school. One day, we decided to get us some free plywood. There was a construction site outside town, see? So we had some beers, then decided to go there at night, steal some plywood, no big deal, right?"

Derek and I nodded.

"So we get there after midnight and the plywood is too big, doesn't fit in the back of the truck. So guess what? We balance it on the top of the truck. Only we didn't have any way to keep it there. So my buddy and I, we sit in the cab of the truck and reach out and try to hold it down with our hands. With our bare hands! What idiots!"

Derek whistled again.

"We turn left onto the highway and the plywood slides right off and cuts my buddy's fingers off and shoots over the truck and hits the road! So we get out and look at it and my buddy's hands are squirting blood and I says, well, heck, I'll get the plywood back and hold it there myself."

Derek shook his head in disbelief.

"You're right. Couldn't do it. My buddy, I ignored him at first but then he passed out so I had to take him to the hospital. Left the plywood there on the highway."

"Did you get caught?" Derek asked.

"Naturally! Next morning the cops were there!" BB laughed.

"Did you go to jail?"

"No. I was seventeen and a half, went to Juvi. When I got out, Dad beat the tar out of me. So I ran away, worked on the oilfield for six months. I learnt a lot from the oil fields.'

"What did you learn?"

"I learned I hated to work in the oilfield. I learned I liked a warm bed and a good sleep and hot meals. So I came back home."

"How was your dad? Was he okay with you coming home?"

"Turned out, he needed me. He had lung cancer and I took him to the VA every couple weeks. I did what I could."

"What about his second wife?"

"Oh, she was long gone. Ran away, I guess. Didn't ask, didn't care. When my dad died, I sold the house and that's how I had some money to party. Ended up in the lake with two cases of beer and all my stupid friends. That's when I lost my arm."

"So there was no one to look after you?"

"No one but Frankie. She found me an apartment. She came every day, even on weekends. She changed my dressings, she gave me my meds, she cooked for me, she got me groceries. But most of all, she *believed* in me. She saved me."

"You're a lucky man," I said.

BB leaned forwards and spoke slowly.

"Doc, let me tell you something. All you need in life is one person, Doc, just *one person*, just one that believes in you. Doesn't have to be your family. Heck, often it *isn't* your family. But all you need is that one person that believes in you and gives you that push and that confidence. When the whole world is spitting on you, when everyone says you're no good, you just need that one person. That's what my Frankie did for me. She believed in me."

"So what did you do?"

"I started a business with what I knew. I knew the oilfield, but, heck, I knew I didn't want to work in it. So I started a business. I supplied water and sand to the oilfield. I hauled away their waste. I brought them food and water. I set up sleeping cabins and toilets. Frankie and I, we set up our oilfield supply company,"

"What's it called?"

"Washington Supply. We got a big old place west of town on the Brownwood highway."

"Yeah, I've seen your lot. You got a big old place! You must be doing good!" Derek said.

"We did okay," BB shrugged. "I drove the trucks, Frankie did the books. We worked our tails off! But I stayed clean, I got me a couple more drivers and a partner and steady and loyal customers so we're blessed!"

BB let go of the wall and grasped Frankie's hand. She blinked at him.

"Never had kids. Maybe on account of her lupus, maybe on account of me. The Lord doesn't make mistakes, the Lord gave me my Frankie and I just accept whatever He has planned for me. The Lord gave me the one person who believed in me and it sure fixed my life. She's all I ever needed."

BB wiped his eyes on his shoulder and looked away. I checked Frankie's vital signs again.

"Her blood pressure is much better now. Her heart rate has settled. How's the pain, Mrs. Frankie?" Derek asked.

Frankie nodded.

"Better," she mumbled.

"Okay then!" Derek whooped. "That fluid bolus did help! Good thing we gave it, right?"

Twenty minutes later we pulled up outside the emergency room at Abilene Memorial Hospital. There were two other ambulances there and a crowd of paramedics. Derek flung the doors open. Two nurses scurried out to receive us.

"Is this the woman with the perforated colon from Hotspur?" they inquired loudly. The paramedics turned around to stare.

"Yes! This is Mrs. Frankie Washington," Derek answered. He disconnected Mrs. Washington's stretcher. "Her vitals are good. We gave her a fluid bolus and got her BP back up."

One of the nurses climbed in and examined Mrs. Washington.

"Her blood pressure's good, one hundred thirty by eighty-five, pulse ninety-two, oxygen sats ninety-three percent. Pretty good for someone with a hole punched in her colon!" the nurse declared.

The paramedics chuckled and crowded around the doors. I flushed.

"This is Dr. Mathur," Derek introduced. The nurse swiveled. She was tall, with curly red hair and freckles. She held out her hand.

"Hello, Dr. Mathur! I'm Mary Lou Sipple, RN. Are you her primary physician?"

"No, I'm her specialist. I'm a gastroenterologist."

Mary Lou recoiled.

"Are you the one who perforated her?" she asked.

I swallowed.

"Yes," I mumbled.

The paramedics gasped and stood back.

We unlocked the stretcher and wheeled it out. The paramedics cleared a path for us, and stepped back an extra foot from me, as though I was contagious. They stared at me with incredulity. I ignored them and ploughed on. Mary Lou led the way briskly and we stormed into the Emergency Room.

"Incoming! We've got incoming! Give me Trauma Room One! We got a surgical emergency! Perforated colon! Perforated colon!" she yelled.

The ER was crowded. There were doctors in green scrubs, paramedics and EMTs in red and black, nurses in blue uniforms and a few policemen and many family members. Two patients were strapped on stretchers, IV poles wobbling and heart monitors in their laps, waiting in front of the central nurses station. Phlebotomists with buckets, respiratory technicians with oxygen cylinders and maintenance staff pushing carts created a throbbing, pulsating nexus.

Mary Lou stopped in the middle.

"Is Trauma One ready? I need it now, and I mean, now! She's got a colon perforation from colonoscopy, she needs to get checked in so get someone from registration and alert Radiology! I called Dr. Morgan and he wants a stat CT non contrast ASAP!"

I marveled at her mastery of the crisis.

"Get Dr. Morgan down here, stat! This is Dr. Mathur. He's the gastroenterologist!" she said.

She paused and lowered her voice a little.

"It was his case," she added.

The audience gasped and stared at me in horror. I opened my mouth but couldn't think of anything to say. An ER doctor waved us on.

"Morgan's on his way! Go to Trauma One! I cleared it. Are you the one who, ah, is involved?" he asked me.

"Yes," I answered miserably, "I'm the one who caused it. Caused the, ah, perforation."

"No, I mean, are you the one who called Dr. Morgan?"

"No, that was my colleague, Dr. Becker."

Mary Lou grabbed my wrist.

"We got Trauma One ready! Let's go!" she ordered.

I used all my pent-up tension to propel the stretcher single-handedly. Trauma One was twice the size of our ER and had smart new monitors, gleaming rows of supplies, and purple, blue, white and black tubes for suction and medical gases hanging from the roof. The walls were studded with instrument pockets, plastic bottles, x-ray sockets and a back-up defibrillator. The floor shone and the room had a reassuring smell of alcohol and bleach. Mary Lou and I quickly re-connected Frankie. BB stood by the door, holding a bag with his wife's clothes and her handbag.

"How are you, Mrs. Washington?" I asked.

"Frankie, I'm Frankie. Hurting a little. Not bad," she answered.

"You're in Abilene now. We're just getting you hooked up to check your blood pressure and give you some extra oxygen. You're looking good!"

"Thanks, Doc. Doc, don't look so worried. Everything's going to be okay," she reassured me. BB called out from the door.

"She's right, Doc. She looks good. And she's mean! You can't get rid of meanness! She's too mean to get hurt. She's going to be just fine!" BB said.

Mary Lou smiled.

"You do look very upset, Dr. Mathur. I'm sure it will be all right. Dr. Morgan is a great surgeon and your patient looks really stable," she said.

"Thank you."

"Hey, Doc!" BB called out.

"Yes?"

"Doc, I may be out of line but I got something to tell you."

I paused.

"Doc, you didn't do nothing wrong. You got her here safely. We appreciate you coming down in the ambulance. You didn't have to do that."

"I wanted to make sure she was safe."

BB coughed.

"We ain't going to sue you, Doc. Don't know if that was on your mind at all, maybe, maybe no. Just want to tell you, Doc. We ain't suing you for nothing. Don't fret yourself, Doc."

I flushed.

"Like I said, I may be way out of line to even bring this up."

Mary Lou looked at me.

"But we ain't suing you, no sir, never. We love you, Doc!"

Mary Lou smiled at me and placed her hand on BB's shoulder.

"Dr. Naunton Morgan is on his way," she said.

Mary Lou checked the IV and drew a blood sample. I sat on a stool and exhaled slowly. I watched the monitors and realized that my own heart rate was also settling down.

CHAPTER 7

SILENT TREATMENT

The doors flung open and a large, solidly built, red-faced man charged in. He wore a cloth cap, thick glasses, green scrubs and boot covers. He snatched up the chart and strode to the bedside.

"Mrs. Washington? I'm Dr. Naunton Morgan," he boomed.

"Thank you for coming," Mrs. Washington said.

"I'm going to examine you," Dr. Morgan said.

He palpated her lower abdomen, then listened with his stethoscope.

"You got a little hole in your intestine down here. Your intestines have shut down. You're leaking fluid into your belly. We're going to fix you right up, don't worry."

I stepped forward. Dr. Morgan continued talking to Frankie.

"I want to tell you something," he said. "These things happen. This is not a big deal. Happens to all of us, it's one of the risks of doing procedures. Your doc in Hotspur, Dr. Mathur here, I know about him. He's done thousands of scopes. You do that many cases, sometimes things don't work out perfectly. Law of averages, it catches up. So let me make it clear: this is no one's fault and it could have happened to anyone."

I was grateful for his statement.

"I know," Frankie nodded.

"Hello. I'm Dr. Mathur," I said.

Dr. Morgan spun around and lifted his glasses to take a good look at me.

"Didn't see you hiding there! Naunton Morgan! Pleased to meet you!" he said. "Good of you to come down with your patient."

"Thanks for helping with my patient."

"Hey, no problem at all! It happens! Karl told me she has lupus, she was on steroids, has a history of complications after hysterectomy. So she's got all the risk factors for a perforation."

"This is her husband, BB," I introduced.

BB dropped the bag and purse and shook hands.

"Hey, Doc. Thanks for helping with my sweet bride. Are you going to fix her up?"

"You bet. I'm going to get a CT scan first, make sure there isn't anything else going on inside her before I open her up."

"Like what?" BB asked.

"Ovarian cysts, adhesions, bladder growths, early cancer, you never know. I want to go in with a road map in front of me. If I'm going to need some help from, say, a gynecologist or kidney surgeon, I want to know all that before I open her up."

BB nodded.

"That sounds right. You go right ahead, Doc. We got good insurance, Medicare and a secondary."

Dr. Morgan nodded.

"Don't worry. We're here to take care of her, no matter what. I just spoke to our radiologist. They're ready for her in X-Ray."

Mary Lou looked out the door. The radiology transporters had appeared. She disconnected Mrs. Washington from the room monitors.

"Hey, Doc! Why the long face?" Dr. Morgan asked.

I shrugged.

"I'm upset. First perforation."

"You can't control everything, man. Don't beat yourself up. Shit happens!"

"I know. This is my first perforation ever."

"It hurts. You always think, I'm going to be so careful, it won't happen to me. But it does. You do enough of them, the law of averages catches up. Doesn't mean you're a bad doctor. You've got to understand. This is a risk we all take, every day."

I nodded and looked away, unconvinced.

"Bad stuff happens. You got to learn and go on," Dr. Morgan said.

BB followed his wife out the door to the CT suite.

"Let's go get coffee," Dr. Morgan said.

"I'm fine."

"No, you're not. You look like a wet chicken that's had its neck wrung and ass whupped. You need some coffee and something to eat. We've got fifteen minutes. I'm taking you to the doctors' dining room."

The doctors' dining room was bright and cheerful. One wall was lined with floor to ceiling windows and flooded the chamber with light. It looked out onto a small patch of grass and two ventilation exhausts. The opposite wall had a soda fountain, coffee machine and a hot buffet. The far wall sported a large TV and had three leather sofas arranged around it. The room had an assortment of small and large tables. A cook was setting out hot food. We got coffee and sat down.

"Coffee's too hot!" Dr. Morgan said, sputtering. "My builder, he always adds a little cold water to his coffee before ever drinking it."

I blew on my coffee and said nothing. I was still thinking of Frankie Washington.

"Hey, look who just walked in!" Dr. Morgan exclaimed. I turned.

A tall, thin, distinguished-looking man with curly gray hair and half-moon glasses had entered the room. His face was smooth and perfect; he looked like a Roman senator. He wore a crisp white coat and crimson tie. He paused in front of the buffet and picked up a plate.

"Hey, it's Marty Wegener! He's one of the gastroenterologists in town. Go and introduce yourself!"

Dr. Morgan cradled his coffee and picked up the TV remote. I walked up to Dr. Wegener.

"Good morning, Dr. Wegener," I said.

He did not turn around.

"Good morning, Dr. Wegener," I repeated loudly, "I'm Dr. Mathur."

He still did not turn around. I turned to look at his face. He was gazing fixedly at the chicken wings and pulled pork and quinoa. I did not see a hearing aid. I spoke a little louder.

"Dr. Wegener, I'm Dr. Mathur. I'm also a gastroenterologist. I'm in Hotspur," I repeated.

Dr. Wegener picked up a pair of tongs and selected four wings. I picked up my pace.

"I've heard of you, Dr. Wegener. I had sent you a letter of introduction and my resume. I'm so glad to finally meet you."

I offered my hand.

Dr. Wegener peeled off some napkins, snatched up cutlery and walked past me. I put my hand down hastily. Dr. Morgan was watching the news. I returned and sat down, stunned and confused.

"He didn't respond. He didn't say anything. He didn't even seem to notice I was there!" I blurted.

"Who didn't?"

"Dr. Wegener."

"Really?" Dr. Morgan asked, surprised.

I nodded.

Dr. Morgan was puzzled. He spoke in a normal voice.

"Hey, Marty! How's it going?"

Dr. Wegener waved back immediately.

"Good! How're you, Naunton?" Dr. Wegener responded.

"I'm great! Hey, how's your hog?"

"Great, man. Just rode it down to Buffalo Gap, had a burger at Perini's. Love my hog!"

"Let me know when you're going next time, we can ride together."

"Yeah!" Dr. Wegener said. He returned to his meal. Dr. Morgan looked at me, puzzled.

I walked over and stood directly in front of Dr. Wegener. I cleared my throat loudly.

"Good morning, Dr. Wegener. I'm Dr. Mathur. It's a pleasure to meet you."

Dr. Wegener kept eating.

"I just wanted to introduce myself."

Dr. Wegener didn't even look up.

"I'm a gastroenterologist as well. I'm in Hotspur. I'm there because I was on a J1 visa."

Dr. Wegener turned towards the TV and bit into another chicken wing.

"You have my resume if you want to read it," I said, finally. There was still no response. My face burned with embarrassment. I returned to my table.

"Whoa!" Dr. Morgan said. "Man, you sure got your ass whupped again!"

"I don't understand what's going on," I said.

Dr. Morgan shrugged.

"Forget it. Have your coffee. If it's cold, throw it away and get another. Nothing worse than lukewarm coffee."

I got fresh coffee and stared at Dr. Wegener. He ate calmly, and wiped his fingers carefully. He added creamer and sugar to his coffee and sipped it slowly. Discarding all self-respect, I gave it one last shot. I took my coffee and went to Dr. Wegener's table and stood between him and the TV.

"Hello, Dr. Wegener. I'm Dr. Mathur. I'm a gastroenterologist in Hotspur. I was the one trying to reach you for the patient who had swallowed a disc battery."

There was no response.

"We contacted you but you were busy, but thanks for, ah, responding," I said, my throat drying up.

Dr. Wegener looked straight ahead but said nothing.

"I just wanted to introduce myself. I had sent your group my resume earlier. I trained at the Royal Cross Hospital in London and at Baylor and MD Anderson Hospital in Houston," I added.

Dr. Wegener picked up his last wing and bit into it. My face burned with embarrassment and I returned to Dr. Morgan.

"That was crazy," Dr. Morgan exclaimed, as I sat down. "I've never seen anything like that!"

I sat down and gulped my coffee.

"He refused to talk to you! He totally ignored you!" Dr. Morgan said.

"Yes."

"I can't believe it. I just can't believe it. I've never seen anyone treated like that."

We drank our coffee in silence. I tried to focus on Dr. Morgan but my mind was utterly confused and upset.

"Don't let it get to you," Dr. Morgan advised, eventually.

I shrugged. Dr. Morgan was grim.

"That's not how we treat people here in Texas," Dr. Morgan said. "I'm ashamed that he treated you that way."

"Forget it. But I don't understand why he's so angry with me," I said.

Dr. Morgan put down his coffee and looked at Dr. Wegener.

"Here's my guess. You're doing procedures in Hotspur. Maybe some people don't like that. I guess they're worried that you don't have backup in case something goes wrong with your scopes. I mean, what if you have a complication? Then you'll have to call over here for help. And they don't want to clean up your mess."

I had an intensely painful spasm in my stomach. Dr. Morgan turned to me and spoke in a stage whisper.

"So why don't you apply for courtesy privileges at this hospital?"

"But I don't live here!"

Dr. Morgan smiled.

"Let me tell you a secret: you don't have to," he said.

"But how could I be on call for the ER? If I get privileges to admit patients to the hospital, in return, don't I have to be on call for patients in the ER? How can I be on call from Hotspur for GI emergencies in

Abilene?"

Dr. Morgan leaned forwards.

"That's the whole beauty of it. You only have to take call if you have *full* privileges. But if you have *courtesy* privileges then you *don't* have to take call!"

"What? I didn't know that!"

Dr. Morgan nodded.

"With courtesy privileges, you can only admit two patients a year yourself. But, hopefully, you won't have more than two complications a year! And you can see *any* number of consults."

I was thunderstruck.

"So if I had a problem I could admit my patient here myself, not have to ask for someone else to do it?"

"Right! But only two a year."

"I would be assured of a bed?"

"Yes."

"Even an ICU bed?"

"Sure. Even an ICU bed, if your patient needed it."

"Let's say I have already admitted two patients under myself. Then what happens?"

"You can always ask me or someone else to admit or take over. Or you can ask for full privileges, but *then* you would have to take call."

"I didn't know about courtesy privileges."

"This hospital is anxious to encourage outlying hospitals to refer patients here. They're doing this to make the process easier for doctors like you."

I was delighted.

"That's great! That would be so helpful! Thanks a lot!" I exclaimed.

Dr. Wegener stood up abruptly, his face red. He crushed his napkins and threw them into the sink. He tossed his food into the trashcan. He glared at Dr. Morgan and strode out, slamming the door.

"Oh, touchy, touchy!" Dr. Morgan winked.

I walked back to the ER. Mary Lou handed me a clipboard.

"I've already done all the paperwork for Mrs. Washington," I protested.

"Oh, this isn't about Mrs. Washington. This is about you. This is your application for courtesy privileges at Abilene Memorial. Dr. Morgan wants you to fill it out right now."

"Right now?"

"Yes. Apparently, Dr. Wegener went straight to Administration and called for an emergency meeting of the Medical Executive Committee."

"What for?"

"Apparently to plug a loophole. It seems that he wants to end courtesy privileges completely."

"Can he do that?"

"He's very powerful. He knows everyone and his group is the only one in town. If he wants the MEC to close that option today, he can make it happen."

"Will everyone support him?"

"The others in his group are really nice but he can be a real asshole. Yes, he can and he will make it happen. Everyone has to refer all GI work in town to his group so they don't want to antagonize him."

I scanned the forms.

"I don't know a lot of the things here, like the exact day my license needs renewal and my medical insurance policy number."

"Write something. Don't leave anything blank. Just write the month if you're not sure if the date and write down the name of your insurance company and where it's based, just write something. Then you can always add details later."

"I can do that. I can write, *call my office for details* or *to be confirmed.*"

"That's cool."

I completed the form and handed it over. Mary Lou scampered out and was back with a stamped receipt and handed me a thick booklet.

"Your application has been filed. Here's the time and date it was filed," she beamed. "And this is a copy of the Rules and Regulations of this hospital."

I thought aloud.

"So now, even if the rules are changed later today, even if the courtesy privileges option is removed, my application went in before the rules were changed?"

"Correct."

"Can they apply the rules retrospectively?"

"That would be a first. It's almost impossible to change rules and apply them retrospectively, but Dr. Wegener is very powerful. All we can say is, we applied before the MEC meeting and when we applied the rules for courtesy privileges were intact."

I thought for a moment.

"You know, Dr. Morgan is going out on a limb for me," I said. "This could hurt him."

Mary Lou grimaced.

"He will pay for this, I know. But Dr. Morgan, he's a good man. I think he took a liking to you and he's decided to support you," she said.

"Even though it means taking on a powerful enemy?"

"His conscience is more powerful."

"He won't get any referrals from Dr. Wegener."

"No, he won't."

"What about the other gastroenterologists in his group?"

"The others are much nicer. They'll probably stop referring for a few weeks then start up again. Fact is, Dr. Morgan is a phenomenal surgeon. People ask for him all the time. Even if the doctors don't want to use him, the patients ask for him."

"But it will hurt his practice, won't it?"

Mary Lou sighed.

"Yes, it will," she admitted.

"So why did he do it? He doesn't owe me anything."

Derek appeared.

"Hey, Doc! We're ready to go back to Hotspur. BB's not coming back."

I turned back to Mary Lou.

"I feel bad that I got Dr. Morgan into this mess. This fight will hurt him."

"He's not scared. He likes a good fight now and then. Guess he likes you. Must believe in you."

"What did you say?" I asked again.

"Guess he *believes* in you. He believes in you, thinks you've got something to offer," Mary Lou said.

Derek clapped me on the shoulder.

"Like BB said. All it takes is *one* person who believes in you, Doc," he said. "It can change your life."

CHAPTER 8

THE MIRACLE OF EASTER

I was pleasantly surprised to get a call from Mr. Samuel Wilson. He was the pastor of the Hotspur Church of Christ and Mrs. Hill's son-in-law. I had my first Thanksgiving dinner in Hotspur in his home, and he and his wife had become my patients. They had recommended me to their friends, and helped grow my practice.

"Sam! Good evening! Good to hear from you!" I said.

"Good evening, Doc. At least I hope it's a good evening. Are you on call?" Sam asked.

"I'm on call all the time. The hospital ran out of money again and I'm covering as much as I can," I said.

Sam sighed.

"I need a favor. Can you please come see someone for me in the ER?" he requested.

"Sure," I said, "Who is it? What's happening?"

"My sweet bride, Bonnie, got into a situation with a convict," he said.

I was taken aback.

"A situation with a convict? What happened?" I asked.

"We were at the Shopping Basket and I was just coming out with some deer corn. Bonnie was in the car waiting for me. Turns out, Sheriff Rasmussen was transporting a convict and had stopped there for something, I don't know what. Well, this convict, he tries to make a run for it. He runs past my car. Bonnie sees him coming and kicks her door open and knocks him down!"

I imagined the scene in the parking lot of the grocery store.

"Then what happened?"

"Bonnie got out and guarded him till the sheriff and his boys got him tied up again."

"How did Bonnie guard him?"

"She pepper-sprayed him. Oh, she had a Beretta."

I gagged.

"She had a *Beretta?*"

"It's a good handgun," Sam countered. "Though I'm strictly Sig Sauer."

"So why do you need me?"

"Well, when she hit him with the door he fell and got some cuts on his face. 'Course his face is all red and swollen on account of the pepper spray. Can you come take a look at him before he goes back to jail? You got time?"

"Actually, this is a good time. I was just watching TV, and Maya and the girls are at the Templars' place."

"Getting ready for the egg hunt? Painting eggs?" Sam asked.

"That's it."

"Well, I would take it as a personal favor if you would come and see this unfortunate gentleman," Sam declared.

"If you forgive me for bringing a bottle of wine to your home for Thanksgiving," I said, "I didn't know then that you were a pastor for the Church of Christ!"

Sam laughed.

"All that's long forgotten. Except by my neighbors, mind you. They've *never* forgotten."

Chad Jarvis Molnyke was thirty, blonde, and scrawny. He sat morosely on the edge of the gurney in an orange jumpsuit, in handcuffs and foot chains, flanked by two deputies. He rubbed his face desperately. His face was swollen and red; his eyelids were ballooned out and barely opened. He had a vertical laceration on the right side of his forehead and dried blood dotted his face and neck. There was a faint smell of pine and herbs. Sam jumped up and shook hands enthusiastically.

"Thank you for coming in, Doc!" Sam sounded relieved. Bonnie beamed in the corner. The deputies looked away.

Simon handed me the clipboard. I scanned the information.

Thirty-one year old white male being transported to Eastland County to face charges of possession of controlled substances and distribution of same. Single. Unemployed. Smokes two packs a day, drinks a six-pack daily and takes no medicines. No surgeries in the past except heart catheterization.

"A heart catheterization? Why did you have a heart catheter study?" I asked. "You're only thirty."

"Don't know," he mumbled.

"Were you having chest pains?"

"Nope."

"Fainting spells?"

"Yeah, I guess."

"But the study was okay? Your heart arteries were okay?"

"They didn't say nothin'. Can you do something about this damn burning on my face?" Chad snapped.

"Simon, get some whole milk from the nurses break room. That's a good antidote for pepper spray."

"Milk?" Chad repeated. "Milk? For my face?"

"Yes. The pepper spray is an acid and milk is slightly alkaline, it will neutralize the acid and stop the burning."

Chad shook his head in disbelief.

"Let's get some labs and an EKG while we have you. Simon, let's also get a CBC, CMP and magnesium and a twelve lead EKG," I ordered.

"Will do, Doctor," Simon swung into action. He called the nurses station, started an IV line, and drew a blood sample.

I examined Chad's face. Close up, his unshaven face looked like red velcro. I noticed an unusual sweet smell mixed with cigarette smoke. I washed his face and forehead clean with saline and peroxide. I soaked gauze in whole milk and swabbed slowly, scooping out the inner angles of his eyes, his ear canals, and the recesses of his nose.

"I'll be damned!" Chad remarked, "Milk damn worked!"

"Don't talk like that!" Bonnie warned, still beaming. Chad glared at her but said nothing. I repeated the soaking.

"I'll be darned!" Chad said, with some defiance.

The laceration was two inches long and J-shaped. There were several scratches and bruises. His mouth had ulcers and his teeth were eroded down to stumps. There were white exudates in the back of his throat, like wisps of cotton wool. There were several scarred red bumps over the upper surface of his elbows, wrists and feet, more on the left side.

"Let's get him to lie down and clean up the laceration with some iodine. He's going to need a tetanus shot," I said.

I completed my examination. His heart and lungs were clear and his abdomen had a tattoo of a lightning bolt hitting a skull. His forearms showed multiple needle marks.

The deputies pulled Chad's sleeve up roughly and Simon gave him the shot. They strapped him to the gurney tightly and curled their fingers under the straps to check.

Simon stuck the EKG leads and got a recording. He showed it to me.

"Doesn't look too bad," he ventured.

"There are some non-specific changes. Nothing too bad," I agreed.

"Could you state what happened? For the official ER record," Simon asked Sam, pleasantly.

Sam Wilson cleared his throat.

"This young man was attempting to escape. He ran from the police car towards mine in the parking lot. I yelled to warn Bonnie. My little Bonnie, my sweet bride, threw the door open just as he came close. Knocked him down! *Wham!* Got him real good!"

The young man winced.

"So he fell down and cut his head open. *Bam!* Lots of blood everywhere, so we figured he needs to be checked out."

I turned to Chad.

"Chad, any other medical problems? Seizures, back pain, urinary problems?"

"Nope."

"Ever had a bad chest infection?" I asked.

"Maybe."

"When was that?"

"When I was in Galveston."

"You mean, when you were in jail last time?"

"Yeah."

"How did you know that?" Simon asked.

"The medical school in Galveston covers the state penitentiary there. It's a big penitentiary, they get felons from all over Texas," I explained.

Simon nodded.

"Have you ever been checked for HIV?" I asked Chad.

Chad glared.

"Yeah."

"And what was the result?"

"They said I got it."

The deputies jumped back.

"You didn't tell us!" one of them cried.

Chad shrugged.

"I ain't gay. They're wrong. Must have got the damn tests messed up."

I sat down next to him.

"Chad, you've been doing IV drugs. You can get HIV from doing drugs. Shared needles get infected," I explained.

Chad looked away.

"You're wrong," he muttered.

"See those red spots? Those are needle marks over your veins, more on the left. That's because you're right handed. You've got needle marks so old, they've scarred. You probably kept jabbing the same spots. You've been smoking pot and then smoking cigarettes to cover up the pot. Maybe you're not doing drugs now. But you've got white patches in your mouth.

That's Candida, a yeast infection. That's not normal. It can be a sign of early HIV infection," I said.

"Candida could also be due to medications," Simon pointed out. I nodded.

"Maybe it's because of some medicine I took," Chad said.

"True, but you're not on any medicine at all. I think you stopped taking your medicine for HIV and it's coming back."

He looked at me and swallowed.

"So what do we do?" he asked, sullenly.

"We need to check your CD4 count. That's the kind of blood cell that gets killed by HIV. We can do it in the blood we just drew. Just need your permission."

Chad nodded.

"Simon is going to have you sign a form that you agree to have your blood checked for HIV," I said.

Chad nodded and signed.

"I'm going to clean your wound and then stitch it up," I said. "Please lie down and hold still."

The deputies inched back closer but didn't touch him. Simon placed towels under his head and neck. I cleaned the wound with saline and then iodine. He jerked when the iodine touched the wound.

"God Almighty!" he cried out.

Sam came forward and put a hand on his shoulder. Bonnie shook her head in disapproval.

"Damn hurts!" Chad complained.

"Yes, I'm sorry. And it's going to hurt some more. I see some gravel. I'm going to clean with peroxide and scrape the gravel off," I said.

Chad howled as the peroxide bubbled in the wound. I folded a piece of gauze and scraped the wound from top to bottom. Small fragments stuck to the fibers of the pad.

"Doc, that hurts! Give me a shot!" Chad moaned.

"Hold on," I said. "I'm going to put on some magnifying glasses and look for small pieces."

"How're you going to get them out?"

"With fine-tipped forceps. Just don't move."

"It hurts, man!" Chad beseeched Sam. Sam gripped Chad's shoulder.

"I know, son," Sam said, "But we got to let the doc do his job. Lie still, son."

Chad whimpered. Simon wore sterile gloves and pulled the wound edges apart. I wore magnifying glasses and searched carefully; I found two fragments. I grasped the smaller one first, for fear of losing it in the swollen tissue. It came out easily.

"That was one," I said.

Chad squeezed his eyes shut and clenched his jaws.

The larger fragment stuck out like a shark fin. I swabbed around it, then gripped it with the forceps, and tugged. Nothing happened. I tugged harder and the skin tented and Chad's eyebrow was yanked up. I eased the tension. Chad blinked hard and tears welled up. I twisted the forceps and pulled again with more force. He cried and Sam pressed down harder, restraining him. I pushed the tissue down with gauze and twisted and pulled. There was a small pop and the fragment burst out, followed by a spray of blood. I stepped back. Simon immediately pressed down with fresh gauze and stopped the bleeding. He pinned Chad's shoulder.

Everyone checked to make sure they hadn't been in contact with his blood. I stepped back and showed Chad the fragment.

"I got a couple out. Looks clean now. I'm going to wash your wound with saline," I said.

"Will it need stitches?" Chad asked.

"Oh, yes!" Simon interjected.

I nodded.

"Yes. I'm going to inject some numbing medicine," I said.

I changed gloves and drew up lidocaine. Chad watched with

apprehension.

"That's a *really* big needle!" Chad complained.

"I'm only using this big needle to draw up the medicine. Then I'm going to change it to a much smaller needle for the actual injection," I promised.

"No, I want a shot for pain first!" Chad tried to sit up. The deputies pushed him down. They had pulled on gloves.

"I've had stitches, son, it's not too bad," Sam said. "Stings in the beginning. Then it goes numb and you don't feel anything."

Chad kept looking at the needle I was going to use.

"Doc, I did some stitching up today myself," Sam said.

"You have animals?" I asked.

Sam snorted.

"Well, it's like this. We got ourselves a ranch last year. We were there this morning. I was shaving when I looked out the window and saw Boxster, my German shepherd, and he was ripping up some little animals and he was all bloody. So I went out to see what he just killed and it was a bunch of little bunny rabbits!"

I injected lidocaine into the laceration. Chad was motionless.

"I suddenly remembered that we had new neighbors and their daughter had just gotten bunnies for Easter. And Boxster had just come running out from the direction of their house! So I gathered up the dead bunnies and took them quickly to the bathroom. I washed them with shampoo and got the blood off. Then I got me some thread and a needle and stitched them up as best I could," Sam continued.

Simon handed me 3-O chromic catgut sutures on a curved needle. I grasped the base of the needle with an artery forceps and lifted the edge of the laceration with another. Sam chuckled.

"Mind you, I just had a straight needle so it was difficult. No fancy curved needles like you have! Luckily, I had white thread. So I kind of stitched them back together best as I could, then fluffed them up with my wife's hair dryer."

Bonnie snorted.

"I had to, precious!" Sam explained, "On account of being our new neighbors and me not wanting to start off with our dog killing their daughter's little Easter bunnies!"

Bonnie shook her head in disgust.

I plunged the curved needle under the opposite flap of skin and pushed up. The tip popped out. I let go of the base of the needle and grabbed the tip with the forceps and pulled the needle out.

"Well, sorry to use your shampoo and hair dryer, precious, but I seriously had no choice," Sam went on. "Anyhow, somehow, I don't know how, I got them bunnies cleaned up and stitched up. Then I sneaked back around the neighbor's house and got to the rabbit cages at the back. Sure enough, they lay there all broken up and open and empty. I put the bunnies back inside and closed the doors, and just shot out of there fast as a bat out of h-e-double hockey sticks!"

"Our new neighbors, you mean, the Traybers?" Bonnie asked, "I saw their truck outside the Shopping Basket."

"Yes, the Traybers. The new neighbors. Well, I just met them inside the Shopping Basket when I was getting the deer corn. Walt comes up to me and he says, Sam, you'll never believe what happened to Tiffany's Easter bunnies."

"Walt was there?" Bonnie gasped, "He knew about the bunnies?"

"Just listen. He comes up to me and says, Sam, we got Tiffany some bunny rabbits for Easter. But they died a week ago! We buried them. Then today we go out to the back yard and *they're back!* Back in their cages! It's an Easter miracle!"

Bonnie suppressed a guffaw.

"What did you say, Sam?" she asked.

"I said, indeed, indeed, it is the season of miracles!" Sam grinned.

I put in the last stitch and Simon snipped the free ends. I surveyed my work, then cleaned it with iodine. Chad winced. He looked morose.

"Sorry. I know that hurts," I said.

"It's okay," Chad shrugged, his voice steadier.

"You might have a scar," I warned.

"Why should I care? I have AIDS. I'm going to die anyway."

For a few seconds, no one spoke.

"Is that true, Doc?" Sam asked quietly.

I hesitated.

"Chad, that depends on your CD4 cell count. If it's well above 500, you're okay. But once it gets below that you're at risk of serious infections," I answered.

"So how many weeks have I got, Doc?" Chad persisted.

"I'm just guessing," I protested.

"Give me your best guess. I know you can't be sure," Chad insisted.

I hesitated.

"If I'm right, and I certainly don't know for sure that you have HIV, just my best guess, maybe three to five years," I answered.

Chad looked away and nodded.

"Galveston doctors told me I had it. Didn't believe them. I ain't gay! Sure, I shot up, who hasn't? I figured you only got AIDS from sex. So I didn't believe them and stopped all the meds cold turkey."

"Chad, you need to get back on the medicines right away!" I implored. "You could pick up a really bad infection."

"And the infection could kill me, I know," Chad said.

"Yes, it could. But if you take your medicines and antibiotics, that will slow down the whole process."

"Just delays it, doesn't fix it," Chad muttered.

"True, but you should fight for time," I said.

"Why? What's the damn use? Die in one month or one year, what's the damn difference? If you got AIDS, you are going to die."

"There's hope. There's a new treatment coming out for HIV. I've been reading in journals that giving three strong medicines together makes a big difference. Actually stops HIV, and patients get a lot better," I said.

Chad shook his head and looked up at the ceiling.

"Nothing stops HIV, Doc. Nothing!" he said, quietly.

"I really think this will work! Chad, do your best to hang in there so we can get you this new treatment."

Simon unstrapped Chad and he sat up. The deputies wore gloves and handcuffed him. He stood up and shivered. He looked gaunt.

"I need a miracle, Doc. A miracle! That's what I need. Otherwise I'm a dead man walking," he said.

"I think this new treatment could be a miracle," I said.

"Are you saying it's a cure?" Chad asked.

"No, not a cure, but the next best thing. Safe, long-term treatment. Some of the medicines haven't been fully tested yet. All I'm saying is that there's a really good chance of surviving if you look after yourself the next couple of years."

Chad pondered.

"I could be normal?" he asked, doubtfully.

"Pretty much."

One of the deputies stepped forward.

"Doc, are you done?" he asked.

"He needs a shot of antibiotics, and I'm going to give him a prescription for antibiotics as well because the wound was dirty. One gram Rocephin, Simon."

Simon drew up the shot. He turned and questioned me.

"Dr. Mathur, what's wrong with his heart?" he asked.

"I was wondering about that. Chad, did you have an angiogram? That's the test in which they poke you in the groin with a big needle and push a long thin tube up to your heart?"

"Yeah. They did that test. I remember they couldn't get me to sleep. I was awake for the whole deal. I watched it all on a TV screen, it was cool,"

Chad said.

"Did they say what they found?"

"Yes, but I don't remember. Some 'A' word."

"Abscess?"

"Nope."

"Atrial septal defect?"

"No, no."

I was puzzled.

"Was it an aneurysm? A mycotic aneurysm?" I asked.

His face brightened.

"That's it! That's the word!" he exclaimed.

"What's a mycotic aneurysm?" Simon asked.

"When bacteria get into the bloodstream and infect part of the lining of the aorta, the biggest artery of the body," I explained.

"How did the bacteria get into the bloodstream?" Simon asked.

"Probably the IV drugs," I answered

"So the bacteria got in because of the dirty IV needles and infected some part of the blood vessel. Then that infected part gets weak and balloons out?" Simon asked.

"Exactly," I answered. "The infected part bulges out a little. I bet that's what they were trying to check. Chad, did they find an aneurysm?"

"Don't know," Chad shrugged. He lost interest and looked away.

"You're going to have to lie down again and pull down your pants, I'm afraid," Simon said, waving the syringe.

Simon gave Chad the antibiotic shot in the buttock.

When he rolled back, Chad's face was flushed and his eyes were red and moist.

"So I guess I'm really screwed," he said, bitterly.

"Those IV drugs really did a number on you," Simon observed. "You got HIV and a heart aneurysm."

Chad stood up shakily. He patted down his hair and wiped his eyes.

He looked like a child, a lost boy. I imagined him without his scarred face and puffy eyes and destroyed teeth and imagined for a second that he was my own son. He was *someone's* son.

"Thanks, Doc," he said, gruffly.

"You're welcome."

"Guess I should have seen the light earlier," he said, ruefully. "Guess I shouldn't have done some of the stuff I done."

"You can still turn things around, son. I mean it. Don't do bad things to your body and take your medicines," I pleaded.

"Doc, I wake up every morning wondering how much time I got left. I won't lie to you. I reckon I'm going to keep doing stuff, whatever shit I can get my hands on."

The deputies looked at each other grimly.

"Listen to me. There will be treatment for HIV. I believe it. You will not die. But you have to look after your health till then."

"How long?"

"One or two years."

"I won't make it."

I grasped his shoulder.

"Yes, you will. I believe in you. You have the will. You handled the pain of the laceration. You got it stitched up and you have courage. I believe you can do it."

"I don't believe that," Chad snapped.

"I believe in you. All you need in life, Chad, is one person who believes in you. I believe you can turn your life around. Just take your medicine and don't get infected or sick for the next couple years and I promise you, there will be a great treatment."

Chad was unconvinced.

"You won't die," I repeated. "Please take your medicines."

Chad shook his head, unconvinced.

"Let's go," a deputy said.

"You can still find Jesus, son," Sam declared, "Let the Lord guide you."

Chad nodded but said nothing. Bonnie gave him a hug.

"I'm sorry for hurting you, son," she said.

Chad nodded again. He glanced at Sam.

"Guess I'm like one of them bunny rabbits you talked about," he said. "I'm dead already, you're just trying to clean me up."

I flinched.

"God bless you, son," Sam wished. "I pray you find hope. This is the season of hope and rejuvenation."

Chad shook his head and walked out with the deputies. They radioed the police car to pull up. None of us spoke. We heard Chad shuffle out. Sam stepped into the corridor.

"Have faith, son, have hope! Jesus came back, son, to give us faith and hope," Sam called out.

The footsteps stopped briefly.

"Then Jesus help me," Chad called back. "Please, Jesus, *help me.*"

CHAPTER 9

CAN'T SWALLOW THIS

"Good morning, Mrs. Gideon," I said.

"What's good about it?" she snapped.

"I'm just wishing you, not stating a fact."

"Nothing good about it. Here I am, hungry and thirsty, waiting for you to look down my throat. How could I have a good morning?"

"You're right. I know how I feel when I haven't had my morning coffee. Let me review your history."

Mrs. Gideon and I were in the operating room of the Hotspur Hospital. She was ready for the procedure to examine her upper digestive system, called an EGD for short.

"You mean, you haven't read my chart yet?"

"I have read your chart. You saw Dr. Becker last week because you were having difficulty swallowing. I've read his notes, but they are a little short, and I need a little more detail."

"Well, I'm not going back to that man," Mrs. Gideon sniffed. "He was back from rehab last week, so I went to see him considering he's my regular doctor and you're my specialist. He upset me and so I'm not going back to him."

"What happened?"

"Well, first I overheard him say that I looked like ten pounds of potatoes in a five pound bag," Mrs. Gideon complained, angrily. "And then, when I told him that I was having difficulty swallowing, do you know what he said?"

"No."

"When I said, I'm having difficulty swallowing, he said, well, it's about time!"

Mrs. Gideon had clearly gained weight, and I suppressed a smile.

"So how long have you had difficulty swallowing?" I asked.

"Two months."

"It was fine before that?"

"Absolutely!"

"So it started suddenly two months ago?"

"Yes. Well, maybe three months, I'm not sure. But I know what it is."

"Really? What do you think it is?"

Mrs. Gideon drew herself up in the bed and motioned for me to come closer.

"Parasites!" she hissed. "Parasites! They're eating me up on the inside!"

"I doubt that, Mrs. Gideon. Parasites don't usually cause swallowing problems."

"Yes. they do. I've been reading on the computer. It's called the kissing bug," she shot back.

"You're right, there's a parasite called T. cruzii, and you get it from bug bites."

Mrs. Gideon arched up in victory.

"I've been bitten by bugs like I was hog-tied in a fire ant dune!" she said.

"But this infection is only seen in South America. Have you ever been there?"

"No."

"Then it's highly unlikely. I've been in medicine almost twenty years and I've never seen a case."

"I have all the symptoms. I know I have a parasite!"

"Have you been taking any anti-inflammatory medicines like aspirin, ibuprofen, naproxen or meloxicam?"

"I've been using Arthur-Right-Is, that new medicine."

"What? That medicine's been recalled! You must stop using it immediately!"

"Well, I haven't been taking it regularly. It didn't work."

"Have you been taking any Vitamin C?"

"No. I mean, I take all sorts of supplements and vitamins, I'm sure there's Vitamin C in one of them."

"But do you take any plain Vitamin C?

"I don't think so."

"What about iron tablets, or any pills for osteoporosis?"

"No. Why are you asking?"

"Because these pills can burn up your esophagus and make it hard to swallow. Your problems started suddenly so I think you took some medicine that hurt your food pipe. There are two others that I can think of, an antibiotic called doxycycline and a heart medicine called quinidine. Have you used those?"

"Never heard of them."

"Any heartburn?"

"All the time. But I take a purple pill for that, and it really helps."

"Do you have problems with solids or liquids?"

"Sometimes solids, sometimes liquids. Sometimes I have no problems at all. It's a puzzle."

"Does food hang up in your throat or your chest?"

"Sometimes it hangs up in my throat, and sometimes in my chest."

"But where does it bother you more? In your throat or your chest?"

"Some days it really hurts in my throat and other days it hurts in my chest."

I paused.

"Does it hang up more often in your throat or more often in your chest?" I asked.

Mrs. Gideon thought.

"About the same," she decided. "Maybe a bit more in my throat."

I reviewed her chart. Mrs. Gideon coughed.

"But I'm not sure. Maybe it hangs up in my chest as well," she added, helpfully.

"Your chart says you have arthritis in your hips and knees. Are you sure you're not taking something for it?" I probed.

"I don't have to, Doctor. I go to a specialist in Oklahoma. He gives me a big shot for arthritis and I'm fine! That magic shot does the trick!"

"What's in the shot?"

"I don't know. Vitamins and supplements, I guess. Dr. Fournier says it's a magic shot and I believe him."

"How long have you been having these shots?"

"Six months."

"How many have you had?"

"One every month."

I stepped back and looked at her carefully.

"Have you noticed that your face has swollen up and become red?"

Mrs. Gideon stared at me, upset.

"Yes."

"Your arms and legs are okay but you have, ah, gained a little weight on your tummy."

"Dr. Becker has already made fun of me."

"I'm not making fun of you. I think you're getting shots of steroids. Steroids cause you to gain weight on your trunk and face but not on your limbs. How's your appetite?"

"Better than ever!"

"Any problems sleeping?"

"Harold says I stay wired up. So does Emily."

"Who's Emily?"

"Emily Youngblood. You know her, you found her colon cancer."

I shook my head.

"I can't discuss other patients, that's a violation of privacy."

Mrs. Gideon smiled patiently.

"This is a small town, Doc. No such thing here!" she shrugged.

"So Harold and Emily say you're wired up?"

"Yes."

"Is it worse after the shots?"

"Maybe. I'm not sure."

"Okay. Is it better right before the shots?"

She thought about it.

"I guess. Harold always has to drag me there. I always feel better afterwards but he says I complain all the way to Tulsa!"

"I think you're getting big doses of steroids. That would explain your weight gain and your face swelling up and turning red, and your appetite and your euphoria."

Mrs. Gideon looked crestfallen.

"He says he's a real doctor. He's got a certificate."

"I don't know about that. It's not good to get big doses of steroids every month."

"Do you think it's causing other problems? Is it affecting my turds?" she asked, hopefully.

"No, I don't think so. But it can cause you to get a yeast infection in your throat. It could be why you're having that swallowing problem."

"Will you be able to tell by looking?"

"Yes. I'll take some biopsies to confirm it, but sometimes it's obvious."

"Can you treat it?"

"Yes. We can cure it."

Mrs. Gideon's eyes shone.

"So I was right! I do have a parasite!" she exulted.

"Well, it's a yeast, not a parasite," I clarified.

"It's a parasite," Mrs. Gideon said firmly.

I decided not to argue further.

"Let's have you lie down and turn on your left side. I want you to bite down on this little piece of plastic. It has a hole in it and that allows me to get the scope between your teeth without you biting down on it."

"So I don't bite your instrument?"

"Correct. And also to protect your teeth from the scope."

Penny appeared with four vials.

"Just got these from the Pharmacy. Two midazolam, two meperidine," she said.

"Thanks. Please draw them up and I'll start giving her the meds. By the way, let's do a finger-stick glucose on her."

"A glucose level? But she's not diabetic," Penny said.

"Not a *known* diabetic. But I think she's been getting big shots of steroids every month from someone in Oklahoma."

"Will that affect your sugar level?"

"Yes. Steroids make your glucose levels go up because they fight your insulin."

I sedated Mrs. Gideon and started the test. I gently advanced the tip of the endoscope into her throat and down her food pipe. The lining was inflamed and there were thick white patches scattered throughout.

"Whoa! What's all that white stuff in her throat? Was she just eating some bread?" Penny burst out.

"No. That's a yeast infection called Candida."

"Is that what you were just talking about?"

"Yes. It's pretty bad."

"How is the stomach?"

I examined the stomach and intestine slowly. I turned the tip back on itself to look up at the roof of the stomach.

"It looks okay. Let's take some biopsies to confirm the yeast infection."

"Do we need to stretch the food pipe open?" Penny asked.

"No. There's nothing to stretch open. She's having difficulty swallowing because the yeast infection is causing the lining of the mouth and food pipe to swell up."

"What are you going to give her?"

"There's a pill called fluconazole. That will clear it up nicely."

"So she has a yeast infection, a fungal infection?"

"I would bet money she does."

"So no parasites?"

"No. Worms or parasites don't generally attack the food pipe. The one she was talking about is only seen in South America, not here in the States."

"She was so convinced she had a parasite. She's going to be disappointed."

"Well, the fungus is a kind of parasite. It feeds completely on the host and provides nothing beneficial in return, so you could stretch the definition," I said.

I biopsied the inner lining of the food pipe and withdrew the endoscope.

Penny jabbed Mrs. Gideon's fingertip with a needle and obtained a drop of blood. She squeezed it onto a test strip. I finished writing my note and checked on Mrs. Gideon. She was stirring.

"Glucose is two-twelve!" Penny reported.

"That's high, especially as she's fasting. That confirms it. She's definitely getting steroid shots in Oklahoma!" I said.

Mrs. Gideon tried to sit up and rubbed her eyes.

"What did you find?" Mrs. Gideon asked, groggily.

"You have a yeast infection," I told her. "I'm going to call Harold and give him the report."

"A yeast infection? That's all?"

"Well, that's good news."

"No, it's not. I told Dr. Becker I had a parasite and he laughed at me. Now you're saying I don't have a parasite."

"Well, yeast is a kind of parasite. It fits the definition."

Mrs. Gideon brightened up

"So I did have a parasite!" she exulted.

"Kind of," I shrugged.

She was so excited she called her husband immediately.

"Harold! Harold! I was *absolutely* right," she gloated, triumphantly. "It *was* a parasite. Go tell Dr. Becker right away!"

CHAPTER 10

THE DOG BITE

It was probably ten in the morning when my nurse pulled me out of a clinic room.

"What is it?" I asked.

"It's Dr. Becker on the phone for you, he's covering the ER," Sharon whispered.

"Karl?" I said, puzzled. I snatched up the phone.

"Hey, man, how's it hanging?" a familiar voice boomed.

"Karl!" I burst out in delight, "How are you? Are you back from your holiday?"

"Holiday? Are you kidding me? I'm in rehab, not on holiday! Not done with rehab, but just another couple weeks, I'll be done, no problem. Hey, I'm actually calling about your wife."

"About Maya?" I said, alarmed, "What happened?"

"She was jogging up in your fancy neighborhood, up on the hill. Dog bit her."

"What? How bad is it?"

"She got bitten on the ankle. Little blood, some swelling. Not too bad, but I told her to come to the ER and I would see her," he said. "I'm covering the ER today."

"So you're here for the full day?"

"Einstein, my rehab is in Dallas. How am I supposed to spend the full day here in Hotspur when I'm supposed to be in Dallas?"

"I'm confused. How are you able to cover the ER here?"

"I drive down from Dallas in the morning, hang around till seven p.m. and then skedaddle back. Rehab's going well, they gave some time off so I could see my family and do a little hospital work."

"So the rehab's going well?"

"Abso-damn-lutely! Real well. I'm almost done, I'll be back home in another couple weeks."

"So you're covering the ER part-time?"

"Bingo! I'm covering the ER part-time, Einstein, seven a.m. to seven a few days. Helps pay the bills. Do you feel threatened?"

I ignored his taunt.

"I'm going to come back and all my patients are going to come back to me."

"That's fine. What happened to the dog?"

"We got it. It's in the pound."

"Is it rabid? I mean, is it showing any kind of weird behavior?"

"Nope, but it did bite the postman last week. He already put in a complaint to Animal Control."

"How do you know all this? Did you talk to the dog's owners?" I asked, surprised.

"It's my parents' dog. They live on the hill, near the Templars. It was their dog that ran out and bit Maya," he explained. "I was visiting them when it happened. He bit Maya before I could get to him, I'm sorry."

"Okay, now I understand. I'll wind up at my clinic and see you down in the ER," I said.

I met Maya in the parking lot and we walked to the ER. She looked remarkably fresh and vibrant.

"I went home and spoke to Anjali and arranged a babysitter. Priya's at school," Maya said.

"Is Anjali with Billie Merryman?"

"Yes. Luckily, she was free. She's the best."

"You don't look sweaty or anything. You had just been running?" I asked.

"Took a quick shower and changed," Maya admitted.

"And put on fresh make-up?"

"I had to be *presentable*," she shrugged.

Simon greeted her with a hug.

"I heard about the dog bite. What happened?" he asked.

"Nothing much. I was just jogging past Karl's parents' house. Their Labrador came running out and bit me on my ankle," Maya explained.

"I've been up on the hill many times. My aunt lives there, just across the street from you," Simon said.

Before Maya could respond, the door flew open and Karl sauntered in. We shook hands and he hugged Maya.

"Karl! So nice to see you again!" Maya said. "Thanks for helping me on the hill."

"Sorry I couldn't get there fast enough. Pardner - that's the dog - is eleven years old and he's getting blind. Don't know how he managed to slip off his leash," Karl said. "Sit down, Maya, let me examine you."

Maya sat in a chair. Karl knelt and examined her right ankle.

"No major damage here. No stitches needed. Will need some cephalexin. Unless the Royal Physician of London prefers something else."

"Cephalexin will be just fine," I said.

Karl grunted. He cleaned the wound thoroughly and examined the bite marks with a magnifying lens,

"Looks pretty darn clean," he said. "I'm going to send her for an x-ray of the foot to check for a fracture"

"Does she really need an x-ray?" I asked. That irritated Karl.

"Just checking everything, okay? Just trying to be safe, covering the bases," he growled. Maya looked at me, then nodded.

Simon took Maya in a wheelchair. After Maya, Karl turned to me, grinning.

"So I hear you really pissed off Wegener!" he said.

I flushed.

"I tried to talk to him, you know, to introduce myself. He just ignored me. Ignored me completely! Acted as if I wasn't there, as if I didn't exist. It was extremely humiliating."

"You reckon he's racist?"

"I don't know. Could be. Or he just doesn't like me professionally. Maybe my qualifications aren't as impressive. He was top of his class at Yale."

"You weren't?"

"No. I was in the upper third, but not at the top."

"Racism is funny, it can be hard to prove. Mind you, I think he's racist."

"Why do you say that?"

"Some of the things he says, and the way he says them. In my book, racism is the selective application of the highest principles and morals based on your color."

"I try not to think of those who dislike me as racist. I don't want to dismiss criticism."

"That's how racists get away with it. Their victims assume it's their own fault."

"Maybe they're not racist, just narrow-minded."

"He's so narrow-minded he could look through a keyhole with both eyes."

I laughed. Karl grinned.

"Anything else happen?" he asked.

"Dr. Morgan made me apply for courtesy privileges so I could admit my patients myself, if needed," I said.

"Yeah, he told me. That's a good thing, but now the specialists that work with Wegener will refuse to see your patients. He's got you on his blacklist, so all his buddies have you blacklisted too."

I swallowed.

"That sounds bad," I said.

Karl went on, sounding remarkably happy.

"Also, I figured you'd want them to offer you a job, now that you're in your last year here in Hotspur. I bet you've sent feelers. But now your chances are zero," he said.

"Thanks, Karl."

"Maybe you should look at Austin or Dallas. There's not going to be a job for you in Abilene. You got to go someplace else."

"I'm looking at doing specialty clinics in other small towns like Bavaria and Winters."

Karl snorted.

"So you want to keep your base in Hotspur and go to places like Bavaria? *Bavaria?* They're so stuck-up! You don't have a snowball's chance in hell there. Forget it."

"I'm not going to get a job with Wegener's GI group. Maybe I can make it work here and go to several little towns instead of going to the big town. The contrarian approach."

"No one has done it before for a reason. It doesn't work."

"So what do you advise?"

"If Wegener doesn't want you in Abilene, go elsewhere, like Austin."

"The other guys in his group are really nice, but Wegener doesn't like me."

"I hope you find a good job in Austin. That's your kind of town."

"What do you mean?"

"It's weird. Austin's weird. You're weird. You need to get out of Dodge and get you to a big city pronto."

"You think I'm weird?"

"Sometimes, yeah. You're definitely a pain in the ass," Karl said, nonchalantly.

I glared at Karl. He was gloating and that irritated me.

"Thanks for your advice. I'll be sure to ignore it," I said.

Karl raised his hands in mock surprise and stepped back.

"Whoa! Touchy, touchy! You are wound up tighter than a two-year clock!"

"Let's talk about something else. I don't want to talk about this."

"I think you're too damn tense. You need to lighten up."

I shrugged and looked away.

"Wasn't there something else that happened?" Karl probed.

"No," I lied.

"I also heard that Wegener wrote a nasty report on you because of that perforation."

I sighed.

"Yes. He did," I admitted.

"What did he say?" Karl asked.

There was no point hiding anything from Karl. He probably knew everything, anyway.

"He said that I should have been more careful given her past history of steroid use. He said the perforation was avoidable and I shouldn't have done it in a small hospital."

Karl thought about it.

"Heck, in that case we shouldn't even give shots in small hospitals. What if the patient has an anaphylactic reaction? We don't have an ICU in a little rural hospital like this."

"Maybe we shouldn't do anything. Maybe we should close down the whole freaking hospital," I said, bitterly.

Karl nodded. He picked up Maya's chart and scribbled.

"Whatever. So forget about getting a job in Abilene, start hunting elsewhere. I know you're not going to stay here," he said, soothingly.

"I may be able to make it work here."

"How? By doing clinics and procedures in a bunch of little towns? Forget it, it'll never work. Get your ass back to Austin or Dallas or Houston, that's where you belong. Or try again in Abilene. Maybe Wegener changes his mind, or leaves, or something."

I waved my hand. I needed to change the subject.

"I'll think about it. I don't want to discuss this any more, Karl. Let's talk about Maya and the dog. Is there a decent chance that the dog could be rabid?" I asked.

Karl shrugged.

"Sure. There's a chance. My parents live on the hill, like you. There's wild brush and wild animals all around. We got rabies in Hotspur County, that's well known. Pardner bit the mailman the other week so, that makes two strikes, so yeah, this could mean curtains for Pardner," he said.

"I hate to do it, but I need to find out if Pardner has rabies. Pardner's showing aggression, has bitten twice, so I think we need to euthanize him and check his brain," I said.

Karl looked away. He shook his head.

"I don't agree. Pardner's always been kind of grumpy. Could be just some doggy dementia, you know, getting old and mean," Karl said. "Kind of, like us."

"We've got to do the right thing," I said.

"Have you ever had a dog?" Karl asked.

"A long time ago."

"They're like family. Heck, they're better'n family! Man, I love that stupid dog. I love that mutt! I don't want to lose him."

I was surprised by Karl's reaction.

"I don't think there's a way out. I mean, he bit two people with no provocation," I said.

"Dogs bite. That's what they do. Pardner's an old dog, he screwed up."

"Twice?"

"Yeah, twice. The alternative is, we could just watch Pardner in the pound for two weeks, and if he shows any signs, then we could put him to sleep and check his brain for rabies."

"No! By then Maya will have had the rabies virus in her body for two weeks!"

"She could start on anti-rabies shots at that time."

"Those are painful! If the dog's brain is clear, she won't need the shots."

"I bet it'll be fine. I bet you, Pardner's fine and Maya doesn't need to take anything, just wait," Karl persisted.

"She would be two weeks late! What if it were too late and the shots didn't work?"

"Try waiting! Take the shots later! They usually work, even if you take them late," Karl pleaded.

"Once you develop the symptoms, you're going to die," I snapped. "Karl, you know that."

"Fine. Okay. Just start the vaccine and the shots right away," Karl suggested.

"Why are you resisting this? The dog doesn't even live with you. To save the dog for your parents?"

"Yeah," Karl shrugged.

"Will your parents be pretty upset about losing Pardner?"

"They've had him since he was a puppy, so it won't be easy. He's part of the family, Sandy. He's in every damn Christmas postcard, smack in the middle!" Karl said.

"I hate to have Pardner put down, but we have to know what's going on. If there's rabies, and Maya gets it, it's fatal."

"You think I don't know that?"

"It's a horrible death, too. There's seizures and frothing and severe muscle cramps. It's agony!"

"I know that, Einstein!"

"You know it's transmitted by saliva. If Pardner licked your parents' hands and they swallowed the saliva, they could get rabies too! Your parents are at risk, too."

Karl was silent.

"Karl, rabies virus lives in the dog's saliva!" I repeated.

"I know the saliva is contagious. I think I know about rabies, Einstein. Tell me, do you know who figured out the rabies vaccine?"

"Not sure."

"Pasteur," Karl nodded.

"Pasteur was a genius. He figured out a lot of things," I said.

"There was a nine-year old kid called Joseph Meister who was bitten badly by a rabid dog. His mother brought him to Pasteur, even though Pasteur wasn't a doctor."

"I had always assumed Pasteur was a doctor."

"You assumed wrong, Einstein. So Pasteur gave the kid a series of shots. He made up the shots from a rabbit he had infected with dog saliva."

"What kind of shots?"

"Pasteur knew that the rabies virus attacks the brain. So he infected a rabbit and made an extract from its brain. The first shot was really dilute, the next shots were more concentrated, twelve or thirteen, I think. Anyhow, the kid survived. It was a miracle!"

"That it was. Pasteur saved the boy and then thousands more," I agreed.

"Hey, do you know what happened to that kid?" Karl added. "He eventually became the caretaker for Pasteur's tomb."

"Sounds appropriate."

Karl rubbed his eyes with the back of his right hand and looked away.

"I don't want to sacrifice Pardner," he sighed. "He's part of the family. You don't have a dog, do you? That's why you don't understand. They're family. Heck, like I said, they're better'n family!"

"I just want you to understand why I'm asking you to do this," I persisted. I was gripped by images of Maya having seizures and frothing at the mouth.

Karl looked at the roof for several minutes. Finally, he looked at me and spoke.

"Okay. We'll let him go. Sandy, I learned a lot in Rehab. I learned to let go. I learned that I cannot control everything and life's not perfect. If Pardner has to go, I understand."

There was an awkward silence.

"Rehab is pretty damn sobering. You know, addiction is like cancer. It can get better but oftentimes it won't go away. Lots of doctors in my program, and some had more than one addiction. One of them, used to be my roommate, had an addiction to porn and alcohol and drugs. Used to play loud Christian music while doing drugs and porn. You know what happened to him?"

"No."

"Killed himself six weeks after finishing the program. Addiction's like a cancer, man, it comes back. Most can't shake it. Many doctors end up killing themselves."

"I didn't know that."

"Most people think addiction is an evil, and only a few bad apples get it. Not true. Lots of doctors get it. Best thing is to get it in the open."

"You've been pretty open."

"If you live in a small town, you better be open. Everyone knows everything, anyway."

"When will you be done with your rehab?"

"Couple weeks more. Then I'll be back full time."

"I'm glad to hear that."

"Really? I know some of my patients are seeing you now."

"They didn't have any choice. Dr. Bulent had a heart attack, and Dr. Anderson had back surgery. I was the only one here."

"Heard you had a love affair with Dr. Ehrlich from Dallas."

I winced.

"Heard you were helping him during a code and he set the poor guy on fire!" Karl said, watching me closely.

I nodded.

"Dr. Ehrlich had cleaned the patient's chest with a lot of alcohol and then, when he gave the shock, he held the paddles just a little off the skin. There was a spark, and the alcohol ignited. That's all."

"That's all? What about you over-riding him and giving the patient a bunch of potassium?"

"He needed it! His potassium was low!" I said, angrily.

"Calm down, calm down!"

"There was a big Board meeting and there was an investigator from Austin. They cleared me," I said.

"And you also managed to piss off old man Rutherford before he died," Karl added, grinning.

"His wife was having a stroke. He wanted me to give her streptokinase to reverse the stroke."

"So what happened?"

"She had active internal bleeding. Streptokinase was contraindicated."

"So you let her have the stroke? Tough call!"

"Yes. Rutherford said he would crucify me. But he changed his mind, he even wrote a nice letter for me to the INS."

Karl whistled.

"You were lucky," he said.

"Thanks."

"Listen. I got to make a living, too. I need to get my snout back in the trough. Just need to get my practice back. Did you get your green cards?"

"Yes."

"Relieved?"

"Incredibly."

"Now you can go back to Houston, you've done your three years here. They need specialists like you in the big cities. Hotspur needs good ole boys like me. Not that I want you to see you leave."

"Now who's being dishonest?"

Karl laughed.

"I wouldn't be too sad, seeing you leave. But no, I don't want that," Karl said, suppressing a smile. "You see, you stay here and be the specialist and I'll be everyone's family practitioner. I'll see all the patients and send you referrals. *Ka-ching, ka-ching!* It could work."

I shuffled uncomfortably.

"I've started doing more procedures in the hospital, both upper endoscopies and colonoscopies."

"Yeah. But you need some help. I saw you struggle with that colonoscopy. We're getting a CRNA."

"A CRNA? Why?"

"So the CRNA can sedate the patient and look after the patient's breathing while you do the procedure. That way you don't have to worry about the anesthesia and you can focus on doing your stuff."

"I can give my own sedation. I don't need anyone else."

"It will help you, man."

"I don't like the idea."

"I knew you would resist. Just give the guy a chance, you'll see it's the right decision."

"You should have checked with me first," I protested.

"You would have said no. You hate to change, you want to keep everything just the same. But things got to change, got to improve. Stop sulking and get with the program!" Karl chided.

"So the CRNA is basically a trained nurse who will give anesthesia to my patients, is that correct?" I clarified.

"Yes."

"But if the CRNA messes up the patient's anesthesia, then who takes responsibility?"

"The CRNA gets sued."

"But I would still be the doctor in charge. I could get sued too."

"Yes, you could."

"You need to let me decide who I work with. I should have interviewed him first."

Karl shrugged.

"You'll like the guy. He's a little rough around the edges, but really good. His name's Hawkeye."

Maya returned in her wheelchair. Simon pushed her in and handed Karl the X-rays. He snapped them onto the viewing box. I walked up to get a closer look and stood next to Karl.

"You're fine, Maya," Karl announced, "No fractures. Unless Sandy sees something."

I traced the lower ends of the tibia and fibula. The bones were intact. I checked the soft tissues around the bones.

"Some swelling but no pieces of dirt or calcium. Looks good," I agreed.

Karl pulled up a stool and sat next to Maya.

"Maya, you have to make a big decision. You could have been exposed to rabies. That dog has bitten one other person. Maybe the dog was just old and confused, maybe he was provoked, I don't know. There's rabies in this county. You could have been exposed to rabies, and rabies is a deadly disease, okay? You could die from rabies!'

"Okay," Maya gulped.

"We can either watch the dog for fourteen days or we can sacrifice him right away and take out the brain and check it for rabies."

"The best way to find out is to sacrifice the dog right away," I urged.

"Kill the dog?" Maya repeated.

"Put him to sleep," I said, soothingly.

"Can't you find out any other way without killing the dog?" Maya asked.

"No, unfortunately that's the best way," Karl said.

"What if I just waited?" Maya asked.

"You're taking a big chance. If you develop rabies, there's no cure. Even in this day and age, there's *no cure* once you get rabies. You will die a terrible death."

"So we really need to know if the dog has rabies. If he does, then what can we do?"

"Then we can prevent you from getting rabies by giving you some shots. I want to warn you, the shots can be painful. But they will protect you."

Maya thought.

"Can we just watch Pardner for a few days? Then if he acts strangely or dies, get a brain biopsy and find out if he had rabies."

Karl shrugged. I burst out.

"No! We can't wait! Once rabies sets in, it's fatal! No one lives, no one! We need to know if the dog has rabies, and we need to know *right away!*" I shouted.

"Thank you for that. I don't remember asking you to butt in, your royal highness," Karl snarled.

"She's my wife! She needs to know. You're not giving her the whole picture!"

Karl glared at me, then turned to Maya.

"I wasn't done, but thanks for doing my job. Maya, Sandy is right. The safest thing is to sacrifice the animal and get it checked for rabies," Karl said, quietly.

Maya was thoughtful.

"I've seen your dad walk the dog every day. I know he's pretty attached to Pardner. I don't want to have Pardner killed. Let's wait and watch him for a few days," she decided.

"No! I don't agree," I protested. "This dog has bitten other people before!"

"It was barely a bite," Maya said.

"The dog is already showing signs of agitation! He had bitten someone already!" I protested.

"Just once," Karl said, softening the news. But I was determined to set the record straight.

"He's bitten one person before you, that we know of. I bet if we asked around, we would find some more instances. Maya, rabies is a horrible disease. It causes weeks of excruciating muscle spasms and seizures. You foam at the mouth, you can't swallow or breathe properly, it's a terrible and very painful death!"

Maya was quiet.

"You could *die* of this!" I shouted.

"Want to change your mind?" Karl asked.

"No," Maya said, "Let's watch the dog. I'll start the shots. That should be safe, correct?"

Karl nodded.

"No! I don't agree!" I bellowed.

"Not your call, Sandy. It's Maya's," Karl said, evenly.

I looked at Maya in frustration.

"This is wrong! We need to sacrifice the dog and find out!" I insisted.

"But we can also find out by just watching the dog for a few days," Maya said.

"Yes, but we're losing valuable time! And what if the dog runs away or something else happens? We need to know right away!"

Maya was not convinced.

"It's my decision. I want to watch the dog for two weeks. I'm okay with starting the shots. I can stop them if Pardner's okay."

I shook my head and pleaded.

"This is the wrong decision! Let the dog get put down!" I begged.

"No. We'll be okay. I know," Maya said, firmly.

"That's wrong! That's a bad decision!" I cried.

"But that's *my* decision," Maya repeated, firmly.

Karl looked at her, then at me. He shrugged.

"Okay. Maya called it. We're going to watch the dog."

I felt defeated and upset. I decided not to argue any further and planned to discuss it with Maya later that evening. I would implore her to change her mind. Karl scrubbed her ankle with soapy water and iodine. There were a few skin breaks.

"Soapy water removes the virus, but let's hope it isn't there," I said.

Karl grunted.

"Take ibuprofen for the pain. I'd say two hundred milligrams every four to six hours as needed."

"I'm going to arrange the vaccine and the immunoglobulin shots," I said.

"You could just wait a day or two, Sandy, I'll take care of it," Karl said.

"No. I can't take that chance," I snapped. "We need to start the treatment today!"

"Fair enough. I'll arrange the vaccine and immunoglobulin. Just give her some ibuprofen, Simon. Four hundred milligrams. Maya, have you eaten something recently, like in the last four to six hours?"

"No."

Simon paused.

"Okay, nix that order. Just go home and eat something first, *then* take four hundred mg of ibuprofen," Karl said.

"Because ibuprofen causes stomach irritation, it's best taken with or after food," Simon explained.

"She better not take Arthur-Right-Is, though," I said.

"Yeah, I heard about that. It got pulled nationwide! Had some additive in it that caused liver failure. I think some folks even died! I can't wait to see the look on that drug rep's face when he comes next time. I'm going to ask him all about it," Karl said.

Maya looked at Karl.

"When will you be completely done with Rehab?" Maya asked.

"Back in action in two weeks," Karl said.

"Great! We should celebrate!" she said.

"Too cold to do a cook-out on the lake. Maybe we could all just go out to that new place in Valera," Karl said.

"I heard it's run by a husband and wife team. They have a fixed menu and they serve food Fridays and Saturdays. It's great food. Prairie View Restaurant, I think," Maya said.

"Good idea. Beats having monkey brains at your house," Karl laughed.

Maya groaned. Simon coughed and cleared his throat.

"Mrs. Mathur, I want to say something before you leave, " Simon said,

"I want to thank you for being so kind to my aunt, Mrs. Hill. She lives across the street from you."

"She's your aunt?" Maya said.

"Yes. She's part of the reason I'm here. She grew up in England, in a town called Coventry. She worked in London during the War. She met Uncle Ben there. She wanted him to meet her parents. She was waiting for him at the railway station the day Coventry was bombed," Simon said.

"When was that?" Maya asked.

"During the Second World War. Coventry was bombed terribly by the Germans," Simon said.

"The city was severely damaged, right?" I said.

"Right. In fact, Auntie lost her sister and parents that night. Lots of people died, thousands of them, that very night. Auntie's home was totally destroyed. If she hadn't been waiting at the station for Uncle Ben, she would have died that night, too," Simon said.

"She's a survivor," Karl said.

"Yes, she's a survivor. There used to be a park near their house, Auntie and her sister used to go there a lot. Uncle made copies of the birdbaths they had there. One of the few things that survived," Simon said.

"I've seen them in her backyard," Maya said.

"Yes. Anyhow, she really loves having you and your girls come over, Mrs. Mathur," Simon smiled. "For hot tea and biscuits and a chat."

"We enjoy going to see her," Maya said.

"She knows she doesn't have much time left," Simon added, "But she's got a positive attitude."

"Yes, she does. I have learnt that from her," Maya said. "I like her approach to life, I listen to her advice."

"I want to tell you that she had a dog that got bitten by some wild animal, maybe a rabid coyote. She panicked and had it put down immediately, and there was no rabies. She regretted that decision forever," Simon said.

Karl was scribbling his note. He stopped and looked up.

"So is there a point to this random half-assed story, Simon?" Karl asked.

"Give life a chance," Simon said. "Whether it's a thousand lives or a single life, a person or a dog, life matters. Thank you for showing mercy, for sparing Pardner. That's what my aunt would have said. Now, Mrs. Mathur, you need your tetanus booster."

CHAPTER 11
SUNDAY, BEAUTIFUL SUNDAY

It is a fact of married life that most arguments are unproductive. Therefore, it's wise to compromise and mitigate, rather than spar and agitate. In this matter, I consider myself rather wise. I find it prudent to permit Maya to prevail, and plan for our family unhindered.

So far, she has done well. We have adjusted. When we arrived in Hotspur, we thought we would struggle through the three years of the contract, but it proved to be enjoyable. Maya taught the girls to read and took them out for walks and bike rides. She cooked a lot. She is outgoing and sociable; she introduced us to all the neighbors. There were the Hastings and their grandson, Mrs. Hill, Mrs. Maureen Giles, the Campbells, Colonel and Collette Pershing, and Dr. Becker's parents. However, none stood out as much as Tommy and Agatha Templar. The Templars went out of their way to make us feel welcome. They left homemade bread and cupcakes and flowers at our door many times. We ate at each other's homes often. We became lifelong friends; we have had every Thanksgiving and every Christmas with them ever since.

Maya took the girls to church a few times, though we are Hindu. She enrolled them in dance and piano classes and Priya joined the local school. Anjali was too young, but Maya signed her up for Mother's Day Out, so Anjali scampered off to the Methodist Church for three hours every Tuesday. Maya insisted that we always have dinner together. If I hadn't finished work at the hospital, I would take a break around six, come home and spend some time, and then go back.

Weekends were sacred. If I was not on call, we completed our chores and housework on Saturdays and kept Sundays to be spent outdoors. Our favorite haunt was Hord's Creek Lake, about ten miles out of town. It offered bike trails and picnic sites. All four of us had bicycles and helmets, and were ready to go by ten. Every neighbor faithfully attended church on Sunday morning. We slid out guiltily, heading in the opposite direction. Our first stop was the Subway next to the gas station on Commercial. There was something daring and inappropriate about sauntering in and ordering sandwiches on those deserted mornings.

We usually reached Hord's Creek Lake fifteen minutes later. Priya and Anjali struggled with their helmets, which seemed to double their height and weight. They clambered onto their bicycles, their heads bobbing dangerously.

"Watch me! I can go really fast, Dad," Priya would declare.

"I go fast, Dad," Anjali would echo.

"Want to race up the hill?"

"Okay!"

"But no cheating!" I would insist.

"We never cheat, Dad. *You're* the one who cheats."

"Dad cheats!" gurgled Anjali.

The races began. They involved going up and down a slight incline, noticeable only when seen in profile, but referred to by Priya as "the hill". The trail ended at the water's edge. The lake was turquoise green, in the shape of a T, created by a stone dam on the stem of the T. Campers and trailers dotted the fringes. Young and old lounged in sagging striped chairs and fanned themselves to the sounds of country music and sports commentaries. The air was heavy with moisture and smelled of cut grass, laundry, charcoal, and roasting meat. An open area was devoted to softball and another lay empty. Beyond the rim of mobile homes and grills and picnic tables and fold-up chairs was a forest of live oaks, red oaks, pecans, junipers and mesquites. Rocky patches, surrounded by cacti and yucca and wild grasses, attracted birds and squirrels. Squirrels darted out from the canopies of the trees and raced up and down the tree trunks. They skipped across the ground, pausing and standing abruptly to reassess. Doves and blue jays sailed and swooped and harassed the squirrels, which seemed to enjoy the attention, racing around in circles with their heads drawn low.

We turned around and rode back on a different path. The asphalt trails were neat and fresh, dusted with dried leaves, twigs and berries, which burst underneath and streaked the trails orange and yellow. We raced around, and the open air and space relaxed us. The girls felt free to pepper me with any question that came to mind.

"Dad, it's so nice here!"

"It's a beautiful day, it really is."

"Are we going to stay here?"

"For right now, yes."

"But are we going to move?"

"I don't know."

"There's a boy in my class called Michael. He said you're going to move to Abilene."

"I don't have a job in Abilene."

"So we're not moving?"

"I did look at a job in Austin, but I don't think that will work out."

"Why not?"

"They want me to join right away. I can't leave at such short notice," I explained.

Priya stopped to adjust her helmet. I dismounted and helped her.

"Dad, why are you so short? Didn't you eat properly when you were a kid?" she asked.

"No, shortness runs in our family. On my mother's side, a lot of people are short."

"Were you poor growing up?"

"No, not at all. I mean, we weren't rich, but we weren't poor either. We had enough."

"But both your parents were doctors."

"Yes, but doctors in India were not rich. All the doctors worked for the government at that time."

"So are *we* rich or poor?"

"We're okay."

They thought about that and seemed satisfied.

"Michael at school said you must be rich because you're a doctor."

"Well, there are different kinds of doctors. Some doctors do make a lot of money."

"Are you one of those?" Priya asked.

"No, he not," Anjali answered, quickly.

"How do you know?"

"No truck," Anjali shrugged

Priya nodded. Then she spotted a grass snake, sunning itself on a rock. We left our bikes and edged closer.

"It's harmless. It's a grass snake," I reassured them.

"Because it eats grass?"

"No, because it's color is green, like grass."

"Are all snakes green?"

"No. They can be any color. Remember, I warned you about rattlesnakes. They are brown and have markings and sometimes they rattle. You have to watch out for them, they're dangerous!"

"You've told us, Dad. Many times."

"Let's go up the hill again!"

We biked up and down until we were exhausted.

Maya caught up with us and nudged us back for lunch.

"Dad showed us a green snake!"

"Grass snake," I corrected.

"Grass snake. And it wasn't poisonous!"

"I don't like snakes," Maya said, stiffening. "Poisonous or not."

"We just have to watch out for rattlers. And copperheads. And water moccasins if you're in the lake," I said.

Maya winced.

"Ugh! I hate all snakes. As I've said before, we need a gun. We've got to have something to protect ourselves, just in case."

"I agree. I'll ask around. We'll probably need a shotgun, not a handgun."

"Why don't we ask the Templars tonight?"

"Good idea. They've lived here all their lives. They can give us some good advice."

"Remember, we have to be there at six tonight. We don't want to be late."

"Don't worry, it's not even one o'clock. We've got plenty of time," I said.

"We will need time. We all need to shower and look our best. We need to look, ah, what's the word?" Maya said.

"Presentable," the girls chimed.

"Yes, *presentable*. I'm not going to the Templars looking messy. I need time, we all need time to go looking our best."

"Let's eat our sandwiches and go to the lake."

"But we must leave in an hour."

We ate our Subway sandwiches and munched the chips, saving some for the ducks and geese. We went out on the pier, and tossed out the crumbs. The girls bubbled with delight as the waterfowl darted and squabbled over Cool Ranch Doritos.

Before long, we were back home, preparing for dinner with the Templars. We scrubbed and polished and the girls tried out different combinations. I retreated to the computer, an old Compaq. I had just unearthed our stock portfolio when Maya called.

"Do you have a bottle of wine for the Templars?"

"Are you sure they drink wine?"

"Yes. Remember when we had them over? They both had wine."

"Do you have anything else? Chocolates? Flowers?"

"No. Just the wine."

"Well, I hope it's a good one. I want them to know we value them."

To Maya's credit, we were there exactly on time. To me, six o'clock had always meant *around* six p.m. In Hotspur, it meant *exactly* six p.m. Mrs. Templar was waiting for us behind the door; she swung it open as soon as we knocked.

"How very nice to meet you all," she exclaimed. "And you're right on time!"

Maya shot me a knowing look.

"And here's Tommy. Tommy, meet the - am I saying it the right way -Mathers?"

"That's very close. Actually it's Mathur. Sounds like Martha, George Washington's wife."

Maya shook hands warmly.

"So nice of you to invite us to your home, Mrs. Templar."

"Oh, you must call me Agatha. We go by Tommy and Agatha. Come in, come in. Oh, my, what darling children! What a beautiful family!"

It was the start of a wonderful relationship.

Agatha Templar was a little over five feet, slender, had short white hair and soft blue eyes. She smelt of floral perfume and crisp linen. Tommy was over six feet tall, had grey blue eyes and was almost bald. Brown and black spots adorned his scalp like camouflage. A trim white mustache covered his upper lip. His hands trembled a little and he walked stiffly. He, too, greeted us warmly.

"Welcome, welcome. Awfully nice to have you. Come on in!" he said.

"We've been planning to have you over for so long! We had such a nice time at your home when you made Indian food, Maya," Agatha said.

Their home was elegant. It was in the shape of a boomerang, with the convex side facing the street. The front door was at the turning point. We entered and walked around a large open copper fireplace behind the front door to enter the main living area. The house was perched close to the edge of the hill, and floor-to-ceiling windows framed spectacular views of Hotspur, Santa Anna Mountain, and the ranchlands. The roof extended over the back porch and protected it from the afternoon sun. Maya loved it.

"I love your house, Agatha. It's so well planned and proportionate," she enthused.

"Well, thank you, Maya. We had it designed by an architect."

"I was just going to ask that question! You know, I'm an architect too."

"Well, how nice! Your kind words have even more - ah - gravity, knowing that you're an architect. Do sit down! Now, what can we get you to drink? We have apple juice and apple cider for the girls."

I pulled out our gift.

"Oh, I almost forgot. I have this for you - I hope you don't mind - it's a bottle of wine."

Tommy and Agatha were pleased. Agatha took the wine and showed it to Tommy.

"Oh, what thoughtful guests you are! Shall we open it now, presh?" Agatha asked.

Tommy nodded.

"Why not? I think that's a great idea. I was going to make highballs but wine will be just fine. Presh, let me take it."

Tommy regarded the bottle.

"A Riesling, I see. You can tell by the shape of the bottle," he said.

Agatha nodded.

"Now the corkscrew is on the upper shelf, by the napkins," she said.

We sat in their living room, spread out over a sofa and four comfortable chairs. An ottoman doubled as a side table.

"We really love it here," said Agatha. "We are so fortunate to have this view."

It was like sitting in a theatre. The land fell away twenty feet from the house, offering a panoramic view. To the left was Santa Anna Mountain, a mesa with radio towers and jagged rock walls, softened by shrubs, cacti and stubby crooked mesquites. Shimmering green and yellow fields stretched from the mesa, in neat squares, rectangles and rhomboids, punctuated by ranch houses, oil wells, ponds, combines, and barns, like a giant motherboard. Highways and roads framed the fields, and a railroad sliced an oblique diagonal through the patchwork.

Tommy brought out four glasses of wine on a circular brass tray. His hands trembled.

"I'm sorry, I hope I haven't spilt anything. Had this tremor for years. Gets worse at times."

"Does it get worse when you're in company? I don't mean to be rude. There is this disease - er, entity, called Essential Tremor and it gets worse the more stressed you are and it goes away when you're not concentrating," I explained.

Tommy looked embarrassed.

"Essential Tremor - that sounds like what my doctor says. Yes, it does get worse when I'm being watched."

"Are you taking anything for it? It's treatable."

"Well, I don't have it that much. Maybe in the future. Wine for everyone?"

Maya raised her hand.

"Orange juice for me, please."

Tommy bowed and retreated to the fridge. As he returned, he continued. "Tell me, how are you liking our little hospital?"

Before I could answer, Maya noticed something near the sliding patio door, partly hidden behind the curtain.

"You have a gun! We were just thinking about getting one," she said.

Agatha nodded.

"It's a Remington pump-action shotgun. Double barreled. We use it to kill rattlesnakes and such," she said.

"I think we need to get one," I said. Tommy nodded.

"Good idea. You never know when some critters will show up in your backyard. We all live close to the brush. If something shows up, you need to get it without having to get close. I recommend a twenty gauge shotgun, double barreled, that would be a safe choice," Tommy said. "Coming back to the hospital. How is it working out for you?"

"It's great," I replied. "I'm setting up the GI Lab so we can do most endoscopic procedures right here in Hotspur rather than sending them to Abilene. That way, I get to practice my specialty and the hospital gets paid a facility fee for the use of the operating room and staff and equipment."

Tommy slapped his thigh.

"Grand! That's grand. Everyone benefits! And how's your clinic doing?"

"The clinic is picking up slowly."

"Bill Hennessy was really pleased with you and was telling everyone in church about you. The Hastings family were recommending you to everyone as well."

"That's nice of them."

"I think you've got a lot of loyal patients here now. You're bound to get busier."

"Sandy saw fourteen patients on Friday," Maya said. "But two of those were in the ER, the emergency room."

"Well, that's good. I'm sure you will be very successful here," Tommy said.

Agatha leaned forwards and lowered her voice.

"May I ask a personal question?"

"Certainly," I replied.

"This is your third year in Hotspur. We realize this is the last year of your contract and you already have your green cards. We all hope that you like it here, and really hope you don't move to Abilene or Austin or somewhere else. We would hate to lose you."

I glanced at Maya.

"That's correct, this is the third and last year of my contract. We have been thinking about what to do," I admitted.

"We hear that you have applied for privileges in Abilene. Does this mean that we are going to lose you to Abilene?"

"No. I applied for privileges in Abilene so that I can have a safety net for my patients, in case I need to transfer patients there. That would only be in an emergency, so I could transfer under my own authority, rather than asking someone there for help."

"Have you had a problem transferring patients there?"

"Yes. I had a patient who needed emergency surgery and the doctor there was tied up in another case."

"Do you have privileges there now?"

"Not yet. I've submitted my application. I'm waiting for their Medical Executive Committee to meet and discuss my application."

"But you would still do all your procedures and surgeries in Hotspur?"

"Yes. I would use Abilene as my safety net."

Tommy cleared his throat.

"Sandy, we worry that you're a specialist. Most specialists live in big cities. Any chance you're going to join the specialist group in Abilene?"

I smiled ruefully.

"I approached them but it didn't work out. I didn't get along with one of them, a Dr. Wegener. The others in the group are much nicer but it would be hard for them to override their colleague. I was offered a job in Austin, but I'm hesitant about it."

"Why? Everyone just loves Austin," Agatha said, bluntly.

"Because they want me to join immediately. They had five gastroenterologists in their group and three of them quit simultaneously. That's a bad sign. Not safe to join them."

"But there's not enough work here in Hotspur to support a specialist," Agatha pointed out.

"I'm planning to do specialist clinics in other little towns. Hotspur would be my base. If the hospital permits it, we can take our equipment to

Bavaria, Winters, and Ballinger."

Agatha and Tommy exchanged glances.

"Well, that might work! What you're saying makes us feel much better. We were worried we might lose you. We heard of that urgent job offer from Austin Gastroenterology Associates," Tommy said.

I was taken aback.

"How do you know those details?"

Tommy grinned.

"Dr. Becker's parents live across the street from us. You told Dr. Becker, he told his parents. They were walking their dog and stopped to talk to us," Agatha said.

Tommy patted Maya's knee appreciatively.

"They were very grateful that you spared Pardner. That was very kind of you," Tommy said.

"That was purely Maya's decision. I was very nervous for two weeks," I admitted. "But the dog was observed and remained normal and showed no signs of rabies."

We ate crackers with Brie and baked sliced zucchini glazed with pesto. Agatha turned to Maya.

"So *you're* not tempted to move to Austin?" she asked.

"We feel settled here. The girls are happy and I've been offered a part-time job by an architectural group in Abilene," Maya said.

"That's wonderful! Which group?"

"The Inigo Jones Group," Maya said.

Agatha nodded in appreciation

"Mr. Jones is very famous. He was the president of the American Institute of Architects when he designed our house and our neighbor's house," she said.

"I didn't know that!" Maya beamed. "I was worried about going back to work, but I feel good about getting back into architecture part-time."

Tommy held up a hand.

"If Mommy isn't happy, nobody's happy. We need Maya to be happy," he said. "We really want you all to stay right here."

"I'm happy to do internal medicine and gastroenterology. I think I can slowly increase my specialty work by doing clinics and procedures in nearby towns. If the hospital agrees to it."

"That's going to be good for Hotspur and all the rural hospitals. I used to be on the hospital board, and I know how important it is to have a reliable hospital," Tommy said.

Priya and Anjali had been coloring and they showed us their artwork. They had taken piano lessons and played for us. Maya enjoyed the baked zucchini and the cheese and sipped juice.

"Maya, don't you drink wine?" Agatha asked.

"I get a headache with wine," she explained. "I enjoy the food, Sandy gets my wine, and I'm the designated driver!"

Tommy turned to me.

"Has modern medicine figured that out? Why do some people get headaches with wine?"

"Actually, yes. The headache is because alcohol releases histamine in the body. In some people, a lot of histamine is released, and that causes a headache."

"What's histamine?"

"It's the same body chemical that causes allergies. So you can actually prevent wine headaches by taking antihistamines."

"I did not know that."

"Of course, taking an antihistamine and then drinking wine will make you very sleepy, so that's not a practical solution," I said.

Maya shrugged.

"I don't miss alcohol. I'm happy giving him my drink and being the driver," Maya repeated.

"What a pair! Don't you have it figured out! But you're missing a great wine! Sandy, you must tell us where you got it."

"From the Wine Store right here in Hotspur. It's a local wine, Hotspur Highlands, and it's been a safe bet for me."

Agatha glanced at Priya and Anjali, busily coloring again.

"And your children are so well behaved, just sitting there and creating masterpieces and reading. It's so nice to see little kids again on this hill. You know, we have grandkids their age."

"How old are your children?"

"Well, Dorothy is thirty-five and Jack is thirty-two. They both live in Virginia and work in DC."

"Washington, DC?"

"Yes. They graduated from Hotspur, both valedictorians, and Dorothy went to Texas Christian University. Jack went to Stanford. Dorothy works for a company involved in cleaning up chemical spills. Dorothy has two boys, Aiden and Avery. Jack is a business consultant. He never married," Agatha said, with a twinge of regret.

Tommy leaned over and grasped Agatha's wrist.

"Well, presh, maybe he'll marry later. You know, just like me."

Agatha nodded.

"Well, Aiden is five and Avery is three. Their dad's name is James, James Cameron. He grew up in San Antonio. He works for the FAA in Washington."

Agatha got up and bustled around, refilling glasses and removing plates.

"Let's have dinner," she said. The girls put away their crayons and washed their hands.

Agatha guided us into the dining room. It was a rectangular room with light green shag carpeting. The long wall in front was flat and bare, punctured only by a small window that faced the road. The window was high enough that no one could see us. The right wall had a sliding screen of carved wood. The left wall sported a built-in glass cabinet, stocked with crystal and silverware. Dinner was displayed on a ledge underneath the glass cabinet. Tommy handed us our plates and urged us along as we helped ourselves to a green salad, chicken tetrazzini, warm bread rolls and fruit.

Agatha stood near the head of the table and directed us with authority.

"Maya, why don't you sit here," she instructed. "And, Dr. Mathur, why don't we have you here, next to me. The girls can be on those two chairs side by side. Tommy, you should sit here, at the head of the table, and I will sit opposite you at the other end."

"I've learned to let Agatha decide the details of our life," Tommy laughed. "I decided to delegate. As you see, she set my glass of water on the left side, because I'm left-handed."

We were impressed by Agatha's planning. Maya picked it up immediately and flashed her approval by nodding exuberantly. We served ourselves and sat down and waited for our hosts. Soon we were all seated. Tommy and Agatha extended their hands and leaned forwards.

"Let us bow our heads," Tommy said.

We all held hands and bowed. Maya and I glanced furtively at the children. They obeyed silently. Tommy prayed.

"Heavenly Father, we thank You for all Your blessings. We ask that You bless this food and all of us at this table. We are grateful for the rain You sent this week. Father, we ask that You help the Mathurs as they stay in this part of Paradise and raise a family. Help us to use this food to strengthen ourselves and do Your work. This we ask in Jesus' name. Amen."

"Amen," we chorused.

"Well, let's eat now! Who's hungry?"

"Me!" whooped Anjali. "Me!"

Everyone laughed. The meal was fun, and the girls regaled Tommy and Agatha with stories from school. Our hosts clapped and applauded.

"I love your stories, Priya," Tommy declared. "Let's have dessert, and then I'm going to tell you a story from my childhood."

Agatha brought out two apple pies and a tub of ice cream. Tommy cut each pie into quarters and added a scoop of ice cream.

"A pie should never be cut into anything smaller than quarters, *never*," Tommy said, reverently. "That is the Templar Rule."

To our surprise, we finished every crumb. Tommy got up to make coffee. Agatha sat him down.

"No, presh. You promised to tell them a story. It's Sunday night and tomorrow is a working day for those who are not retired. So please start your story, and I will get the decaf."

Tommy shrugged and sat down again.

"Priya and Anjali, I wanted to tell you a story about me and my little brother, Hap. When we were growing up, I think I was eleven and Hap was nine, Mother had a little vegetable patch in the back, and she loved growing her own zucchini and squash and collard greens. But we had a problem. Father had a donkey, and that donkey would go and eat up all of Mother's vegetables. Hap and I, we built her a fence, but that donkey would get through it on Sunday mornings when we were away at church. He would tear up all the vegetables and Mother would be so upset! So Hap and I, I guess we were a little older than you, we decided to do something about it."

"You wanted to stop the donkey eating the vegetables?" Priya asked.

"Yes, exactly. We tried adding more wire to the fence, but it didn't help. We tried barbed wire, but that didn't work either. So we figured we had to do something different. Something new," Tommy explained.

Agatha set out four cups for coffee.

"We had heard of an electric fence, you know, one that had copper wires with a little electricity. We ordered it from Sears, and we set it up, you know, set up an electric fence around Mother's vegetables. The problem was, we needed a small battery and we didn't have any. So we hunted around and found a car battery instead. Now, the car battery was much more powerful than the one we were supposed to use, but that's all we could find. Hap and I hooked it up on Sunday morning before we left for church, and luckily that morning, services were short. As soon as we got back, Hap and I dashed off to the vegetable patch. Sure enough, the donkey was there. Hap and I hid behind nearby trees and watched."

Agatha poured the coffee and nodded sagely.

"Well, the donkey seemed to sense that there was something different. It inspected the wires. It sniffed the air. It turned its head this way and that, and then seemed to give up. It backed up a little bit and Hap and I figured that nothing was going to happen."

Tommy took a long draught of coffee. Priya and Anjali were completely engaged.

"Suddenly, the donkey changed its mind. It went back to the fence and looked at the new wires. It stood still for a few minutes, then it took out its big grey tongue and wrapped it around the wire. There was this burst of blue flame from his mouth and he jumped up two feet in the air! All four legs went stiff and moved straight out like sticks! He broke wind so loudly, *boom*, they heard it indoors! The donkey fell hard on his belly, *wham*, his legs still sticking straight out like sticks."

"Wind broke?" Anjali asked, amidst the guffaws.

"It means the donkey farted," Priya explained.

Anjali burst into peals of laughter.

"The donkey farted! The donkey *farted!*" she repeated, rocking with laughter.

"I don't know if she understood the rest of your story, precious, but she loved the punch line," Agatha smiled.

"That donkey never touched Mother's vegetables again," Tommy ended, proudly.

Agatha would not let us help clean up. She insisted she would get help the next day. We thanked them and walked home in the brisk night air. The girls kept giggling. They bathed quickly and changed, and were soon in bed. Maya and I sat on the floor outside their room. The house was dark, and finally there was silence. We listened for the rustling to slow down and cease and soon heard the faint flutes of sleep.

As we got up, Maya leaned forwards.

"*This* is the life I always wanted in America," she whispered.

CHAPTER 12

HAWKEYE

"Yo, Einstein! I got news for you."

I looked up.

"I see you sitting in the office and moping. Pathetic! Are you still mourning that complication you had?"

I shrugged.

"That nasty SOB wrote you up for the perforation, so what? Shit happens. Mistakes happen."

"I know."

"The family loves you! Word is, they're not going to sue you."

"I know. But I should have known better."

Karl snorted.

"You are making the whole darn office sad and dull. Stop it!"

"I'll get over it."

"Look at the bright side of things. Mrs. Washington made it through the surgery, didn't she?"

"Yes."

"Sure she ain't going to sue you?"

"No."

"Her one-armed husband isn't going to beat you up?"

"No."

"So, good deal! You learnt something, the patient's good, the family loves you, you riding in the ambulance and all. You just *had* to ride with them, didn't you?"

"I was really worried about her."

"You are a real suck-up, you know that?"

"I do what I'm comfortable doing."

"I mean, which doctor holds your hand and kisses your feet all the way to Abilene? You must have been shit scared."

"I was worried for her, I didn't want her to collapse on the way to Abilene."

"She wasn't going to collapse! She was stable," Karl scoffed.

"I don't know, Karl. I've never had a perforation before. Maybe you know better?"

Karl smiled and took a long drag of his coffee.

"Oh, oh, I touched a nerve! Tracy, did you see the coffee deal I got him? No? Hold it up, man!"

I sighed and held up my silver coffee cup.

"What does it say, Dr. Mathur?" Tracy asked, peering from her desk.

Karl grinned and looked at me, daring me.

"Shit specialist," I announced.

"Oh, my word! Dr. Mathur! Throw it away!" Tracy was aghast.

"Keeps me modest," I said.

"It's awful!" she declared.

I shrugged. Karl guffawed.

"No, it's not. Tracy, you are a painful prune. Go back to your work," he laughed.

"You started it," Tracy protested.

"And now I'm ending it. Go back to work. If I need your advice, I'll give it to you."

Tracy shook her head and turned away.

"So, Einstein, I have news for you. I spoke to my friends in Abilene and Wichita Falls and San Angelo. I told them you need a CRNA to help you with your procedures."

"No, I don't! I'm perfectly fine! I can give sedation by myself, and I don't need someone else to do something I can do myself!"

"Hey, relax, man. You are so uptight! I told you about this when Maya was in the ER with the dog bite deal. Look, you're doing the scope. So, do the scope. That's what you are trained to do. Let someone else sedate your patient and look after the airway and breathing and oxygen and all."

"I *can* do it myself."

"Hey, I *can* do heart surgery, man! But I can't do it *well*. You can't do anesthesia well. Let an expert do it for you."

"But I was trained to give sedation," I protested.

"Twain said, I never let my schooling interfere with my education," Karl quoted.

I laughed.

"So wouldn't it be great if you could just focus on the patient and the scope and do your endoscopy and not have to worry about the patient's oxygen level dropping or EKG changing, or some screw-up with the heart rate, or secretions?"

I paused. Karl was convincing.

"Hey, what? Am I right or am I right?"

"You have a point," I admitted.

"I have a point? You're the Royal physician of Texas and surely the Queen of England is pissed with you for perforating a patient, fortunately not one of Her Majesty's subjects. You aren't going to do a thing about it?"

"I said, I see your point."

"You're not going to be on the Queen's honors list."

"I know."

"She's not inviting you to Buckingham Palace for dinner and a movie and a cuddle."

"I know."

"She's not even inviting you for tea! Her supreme highness is *so* pissed!" Karl said in a high falsetto, waving his hands airily.

"So you think I should have a CRNA who would give anesthesia and I would be free to just do the endoscopy?"

Karl beamed.

"Bingo! See, Tracy, I told you he wasn't a complete idiot!"

"Can we afford it?" I asked.

"See, that's the beauty of the whole deal. The CRNA would bill insurance separately. They get paid as a provider by the insurance directly, and we don't have to pay them anything."

"So it doesn't cost the hospital anything?"

"Not a dime. They get paid by the patient's insurance."

"The CRNA is a nurse anesthetist. So who would be the doctor in charge? Who would be responsible if something went wrong?" I asked.

"I love it, you always think of the worst situations first. You can have an anesthesiology doctor in charge, or you could be the one in charge."

"I want there to be an anesthesiology doctor to be in charge."

"Yeah, and I want to be the Shah of Iran. Ain't happening, Einstein. We are really lucky to get a CRNA to even come to Hotspur. We're not getting anyone with a doctor attached."

"I don't want to take on any more risk."

"There's more risk if you keep giving anesthesia yourself. What if your patient had a different complication, maybe a lung complication like pneumonia?"

"You mean, they had a colonoscopy and then developed lung problems, like pneumonia or bronchitis?"

"Yes, o mighty genius."

"So a CRNA could have prevented that?"

"Exactly. By looking after the airway. While you're busy snipping off polyps, you want someone else watching out for the airway, checking the vital signs, making sure your sweet little lady or big old boy isn't fixing to croak."

I thought about that.

"I understand. If we can get someone who's decent, then I can focus on my work and not worry about the patient waking up or getting agitated," I said, slowly.

"Right! And I've got someone lined up for you. Someone who's pretty dang decent!"

"Already?"

"Yep. His name's Cutter McCullough. Goes by Hawkeye. He's a little bit rough around the edges, but I think you and him'll get along real well."

"Maybe I should meet him first."

"Maybe you're fixing to meet him pretty darn soon! I got a guy downstairs, Castenada, heavy smoker, chronic bronchitis and COPD, came in with a hemoglobin of nine."

"Nine! That's pretty low for someone with lung problems like COPD."

"I know that, Einstein. Patients with lung problems have a hard time getting oxygen so they make more hemoglobin to grab as much oxygen as they can with every breath. So lung patients usually have a high hemoglobin level. It's called secondary polycythemia."

"So his normal hemoglobin should be fourteen or fifteen."

"Yes, Majesty. So his hemoglobin of nine is a big deal. So will your lordship please scope him and check him for an ulcer?"

"Any signs of bleeding like passing bright red blood or black tarry stools? Or spitting up blood?"

"He threw up some blood this morning but hasn't since then. Had one black stool."

"Any ibuprofen or naproxen or similar meds?"

"He lives on ibuprofen. Takes six to eight a day for back pain. I stopped his Arthur-Right-Is."

"Good! Don't give him Arthur-Right-Is. That's a dangerous medicine."

"Hasn't it been recalled?"

"Yes, it has. I'll go see him. Is there any family in the room?"

"His wife Prunella. I already told Penny you were going to scope him and I asked Cutter to be here for the case."

"Where does Cutter live?"

"Out in the sticks. Place called Rising Star."

"I've driven through it on the way to Dallas. Small pharmacy, near the Dairy Queen."

"You're so brilliant, doctor, you're God's gift to humanity, you know every trivial thing. Now finish your coffee and go see my patient. Name's Dominic Castenada, sixty-four years old."

An hour later, Penny and I were rolling Mr. Casteneda into the Operating Room. A bald, stocky man was waiting there for us. As we entered, he heaved himself off his stool and glared at us. He was unshaven and looked tired. His eyes were slits and his nose and cheeks were fleshy. He wore light green scrubs that were labeled *San Angelo Memorial Hospital*.

"So this is the patient?" he snapped.

"Yes."

"Certainly took your time. What's the matter, lost your way in this big hospital?"

I was irritated.

"The elevator is slow. It also took time to get consent. Who are you?" I said, matching his tone.

"I'm Hawkeye McCullough. I'm your new CRNA. And I'm not pleased to be here, just for the record."

We rolled into the room, aligned the patient's bed, and brought his head near the anesthesia machine. Penny was not amused.

"If you're not happy to be here, Mr. Hockey, then why are you here?" Penny asked, curtly.

"Because I'm going through a divorce and can't stand to be in San Damn Angelo so I have to live with my parents in Rising Damn Star and I need the money and you can't get anybody else and no one else will take me, okay?" Hawkeye spat out.

"Well, we really don't want you here then. Maybe you can forget about us and go back, Mr. Hockey," Penny said.

"It's Hawkeye, not Hockey. And do you think I would be here if anyone else would take me?"

"This is a nice hospital. The people are good people. We want decent hospital staff who are happy to be here, not an old sourpuss."

"You're stuck with me, okay, sister? No one else will come here."

"We were doing just fine. Maybe you can take that rotten attitude of yours and stick it up somewhere else."

Hawkeye leered.

"That's what she said," he quipped.

Penny was horrified.

"What? How *dare* you talk like that! That's no way to speak in front of a lady."

"I don't see no lady."

"Take it back! Take it back!" Penny cried.

Hawkeye rolled his eyes.

"How? How can I take it back? I just said it and it's done. Over! Can't take it back."

Penny set the endoscope down on top of the cart. Her face remained flushed.

"Don't you ever, *ever*, ever talk to me like that again!" she hissed.

Hawkeye shrugged and looked away. Penny cleared her throat and crossed her arms.

"You're touchy, sister," Hawkeye said. "I don't know if we're going to get along."

"Let's get the patient ready," I said.

We connected Mr. Casteneda to oxygen, applied the heart leads, and strapped on a blood pressure cuff. Hawkeye slipped an oximeter clip on his fingertip.

"Are you the doctor?" Hawkeye asked me.

"Yes. I'm Dr. Mathur. Dr. Becker told me about you."

"Call me Hawkeye. Pleased to meet you. Kind of. Sorry, I'm a little short, didn't sleep much last night. So what's the story about this guy?"

"He's sixty-four, married, has chronic obstructive pulmonary disease and presented with fatigue. Vomited blood earlier today. He was found to have a hemoglobin of nine grams percent."

"Okay, So you think that he's lost blood from his stomach, so we're fixing to do an upper scope. Right?"

"Right."

"I got a list of his meds. Mr. Castenada, you take diltiazem for your high blood pressure and allopurinol to prevent gout. Do you still smoke a pack of cigarettes daily?" Hawkeye asked.

"Half a pack now. I cut down,"

"You need to quit completely, man. It's killing you!"

"Yeah, I know," Mr. Castenada mumbled.

"You're also taking two inhalers for your COPD, and you use a CPAP machine at night for your sleep apnea. Ever had anesthesia problems after surgery or procedures?"

Mr. Castenada nodded.

"Yeah, sometimes it's really hard to wake me up and my oxygen goes way way down."

Hawkeye scowled.

"Just what we need. A bad airway. Just a little bit of Versed could stop his breathing, just knock the tar out of him. Great case, Doc."

"That's why we have you, Hawkeye. You're going to watch over his airway and look after his breathing," I tried to sound reassuring.

"With what? I got nothing. Nothing! This machine's so old it belongs in the Smithsonian. Heck, does it run on electricity or gas or mule? It's so old, they should have destroyed it. Guess I'm going to have to bag him by hand to keep him breathing."

Mr. Casteneda was alarmed. He tried to sit up.

"Doc, if this isn't safe, then don't do it," he said.

"Hey, relax, Mr. C," Hawkeye said. "All you need is a little bitty procedure called upper endoscopy. I can do them anywhere. Now if you needed your appendix taken out or your gallbladder cut out, I would tell you to go to San Angelo, but you're not having anything major."

Mr. Casteneda was unconvinced.

"Doc, let's reschedule this," he said.

"Mr. C, I'm sorry I was mouthing off. I apologize. Shouldn't have scared you. Relax, you're going to be just fine. When was the last time you ate or drank anything?" Hawkeye said.

Mr. Castenada looked at him.

"Really? You mean it? It's safe to do this?"

"Yeah. I mean it. I got years and years of experience. I can tell when someone is going to be okay and when he ain't. You, sir, are going to be just fine," Hawkeye said. "When was the last time you ate or drank anything?"

Mr. Casteneda paused.

"Last night, around six."

Hawkeye nodded. He rubbed Mr. Casteneda's shoulder reassuringly and tightened the nasal tubing and turned up the oxygen.

"I'm cranking up the oxygen to six litres, okay? You, nursy, check the blood pressure cuff and heart leads."

"My name is Penny. I would appreciate you addressing me as Nurse Penny."

"Suck it up, buttercup," Hawkeye said.

Penny took a step back and pointed to herself.

"Nurse Penny," she repeated, coldly.

Hawkeye waved his hands and shook his head.

"Alright then. Nurse Penny, would you kindly get off your high horse and look after the patient?" he said, in a softer voice.

Penny started to say something, then stopped. Hawkeye lifted up the long oxygen tubing and waved the loops in her face.

"That's a crazy long oxygen tubing. Don't you have anything shorter? It's so long, it's looping up and lying on the ground," Hawkeye complained.

"No. Take it or leave it, Mr. Hockey."

Hawkeye examined the end of the tube and felt the oxygen whistling past with his fingertips. He dropped the plastic tubing on the floor.

"Fine. So long as there's oxygen coming out this end, I guess I'm okay. You ready, Doc?"

"Yes. Penny, do we have cautery?"

"Yes, Doc."

"What about ten cc of adrenaline for injection?"

"I have it drawn up, and the injection catheter has been primed."

"Great. Mr. Casteneda, do you have any questions?"

Mr. Castenada looked uncertain.

"He doesn't have any questions, Doc, other than when are you going to ever get started?" Hawkeye said.

I glared at him. I tried to think of something to say.

"Starting sometime this year would be nice," Hawkeye went on, unfazed.

We turned the patient onto his left side. Penny placed a bite block between his teeth.

"This is a bite block," she explained. "It's a little plastic donut with a hole in the middle. You bite down on it and we put the scope in through the hole."

"So that I don't bite down on your scope instrument?"

"That's right."

Mr. Casteneda nodded, and Penny strapped the device into place.

"Mr. C, you're going to feel a little burning in your vein now," Hawkeye warned. "I've started giving you some lidocaine to numb the vein. Then I'll give you the real stuff, propofol! It hurts as it goes in."

Mr. Casteneda's eyes widened and he shuddered.

"It works pretty fast. It won't hurt for long. Just take some deep breaths," Hawkeye said.

Within seconds, Mr. Casteneda was asleep.

"Go ahead, Doc," Hawkeye urged. "Hurry up! He's kind of brittle."

Penny turned the lights out. The screen lit up and showed the view from the tip of the endoscope. I quickly checked the instrument and placed the tip in Mr. Casteneda's mouth. I slid it over the tongue and into the pharynx. Mr. Castenada did not protest.

"Whoa, look at those vocal cords! They're pretty boggy!" Hawkeye said.

"He must be aspirating stomach acid at night."

"He's got sleep apnea and he says he uses his mask. The positive pressure mask should push fluids down and keep them in his stomach, Doc."

"I know. Yes, He's got sleep apnea but I bet he's not using his mask properly."

"Just on the basis of the vocal cords, you're saying that?"

"The vocal cords are clearly swollen. I just saw them. They wouldn't be like that if he was using his mask properly."

"Like Groucho Marx said, who are you gonna believe, me, or your own eyes?" Hawkeye chuckled.

I passed through the food pipe.

"Food pipe okay?" Penny asked.

"Yes, the esophagus is clear," I said.

"What were you looking for?" Penny asked.

"Any bleeding, swollen veins called varices, ulcers, and cancer. But now we're in the stomach and we have a problem. There's a lot of water and bile here."

Hawkeye swore.

"Suck it out of him quickly, Doc! He might upchuck all that corruption into his lungs! He could get pneumonia!"

"Yes, I know. Raise his head up. Penny, turn up the suction!"

I moved the tip of the scope around the stomach and suctioned for several minutes.

"He had a lot of liquid in his stomach, the canister's pretty full already," Penny said.

The canister had filled up with thick green fluid streaked with mucus and blood.

"Now I've suctioned out the stomach, I'm going to inflate it with air,"

I said.

Before I could introduce air, Mr. Casteneda started coughing. He retched and stomach contents burst onto the pillow and blankets. Hawkeye snatched a suction catheter and inserted it into our patient's mouth and started sucking out thick stringy green residue.

"I can stand blood but I can't stand this thick foul stomach crap," Hawkeye declared, shuddering. "It's disgusting!"

I shrugged. I inflated air and inspected the stomach, looking for an ulcer. Hawkeye groaned as Mr. Castenada heaved and another wave of greenish brown liquid spurted onto the pillow.

"He might need intubation," I said.

"Take another look. If there's any fluid left then I will put a tube in his lungs."

I pumped gas into the stomach. It distended slowly. There was no more liquid.

"What made you go into this awful specialty, gastroenterology?" Hawkeye wondered.

"There was an opening," I answered, without thinking. Hawkeye laughed.

I realized what I had said, and at that moment I saw the source of the bleeding. There was a stomach ulcer in the lowest part of the stomach, the size of a quarter, and twice as deep. It was covered with black congealed clot, and wisps of bright red blood oozed from the edges.

"Okay, I've found the problem! He's got a big ulcer at the lower end of his stomach," I said.

I cleared away the last dregs of liquid and injected more air.

"It's still bleeding, Doc," Penny said, fearfully.

"Yes, and it's located in the lower end of the stomach, called the antrum. This is where the stomach narrows down and the ulcer has scarred up the whole area. That's why there was so much water and bile and blood collected here."

"Because it couldn't drain out?"

"Exactly."

An alarm went off suddenly.

"His oxygen's going down!" Hawkeye hollered.

Penny moved out of the corner and came closer to Hawkeye.

"Can I help you?"

"No! I can handle it!"

"You want me to hold his head back? Extend his neck?"

"No! I can handle it!"

"I'm only trying to help."

"Did I ask for your help?"

Penny shook her head. Nevertheless, she remained standing by Hawkeye.

"Did I ask for your help? Did I say, help me? No. No! I *don't* need your help, okay?"

Hawkeye straightened Mr. Casteneda's neck and pulled his head back forcefully, straightening out the airway. He suctioned vigorously.

"His oxygen's coming back up, that's good," Penny said.

"I told you, I can handle it! I don't need your help, okay?"

"Okay," Penny said, crestfallen.

"Go back to your corner and stay there! Maybe Dr. Mathur needs you, but I don't."

Penny retreated in the dark and stood behind me.

"Penny, give me a snare. I'm going to peel the clot off the ulcer."

"You're going to *remove* the clot?" Penny was incredulous.

"Yes. I need to see if there's a blood vessel hidden underneath. If there is, then I need to cauterize it."

"Will it be safe? I mean, what if he starts bleeding when you pull the clot off?" Hawkeye asked.

"There's always that risk. But at least, I have you to help watch the airway and manage the patient."

Hawkeye gulped.

"Yeah," he agreed. "I guess you know we got no back-up, here."

"Doc, is it safe to pull the clot off the ulcer?" Penny asked.

"We have to see if there's an exposed vessel hidden underneath," I repeated.

"Yes, but he's not bleeding right now. Shouldn't we just wait and give it time to heal?"

"I understand but this question has been studied. We *need* to look. That's the right thing to do."

"In Houston, maybe. I just don't think it's a good idea in Hotspur."

I grabbed the snare and advanced it through the endoscope. It appeared on the screen.

"Uh huh. Open the snare," I ordered.

"Doc, are you sure?"

"Open the snare, *please*. Thank you. I'm grasping the corner of the clot and I'm tugging gently."

"Be gentle! Be gentle, Doc!" Penny urged. "We're out here in the middle of nowhere and you're stripping a blood clot off an ulcer and you might make it break loose and it could start bleeding big time!"

"I understand that, Penny."

"Just saying."

I lifted up the corner. I had pulled a third of the clot off when there was a spurt of blood.

"Yow! Doc! Stop it!" Hawkeye yelled.

I stopped and held my breath. There was no further bleeding.

"I can't believe you're not getting the heck out of there!" Hawkeye said.

"There was some blood trapped underneath. Let's see what happens," I said.

"On your head be it!" Hawkeye declared, shaking his head. "I say, get the heck out of there! Put the dang clot back!"

I pulled the corner gingerly and lifted up. I changed my angle and twisted around.

"It's like you're pulling a shroud off a dead body!"

The oxygen alarm went off again.

"No! No! What's wrong with this guy? His lungs are the worst I've ever seen!"

Penny moved forward, then froze. I looked at her and shook my head. She moved next to Hawkeye and stared at him.

"Don't even say it," he snarled. "*Don't* offer to help. I swear, I'm so close to screaming!"

Penny stayed stubbornly in place by the patient's side. Hawkeye again suctioned the throat and changed to a facemask. I increased the oxygen and we watched the monitor, transfixed. Penny refused to go back into her corner.

"Okay, his oxygen's coming up. Penny, stay where you are. I might need your help, maybe. Just don't say anything, okay?" Hawkeye snapped.

Penny nodded meekly, but smiled.

"I knew you would need my help," she said.

That infuriated Hawkeye.

"Go ahead, Doc, I can handle this. And you know what, Nurse Penny? I don't need your help!" Hawkeye snarled. "Go back to your damn corner. You're crowding me."

Penny's face fell. She shuffled back. I gently pulled the clot off the ulcer. No one breathed. I washed the ulcer base clean with a jet of water.

"The base is clean. No vessel," I declared.

"Hurry up, Doc. I don't know why, but his dang oxygen is dropping again. Hurry up!" Hawkeye cried.

"At least the ulcer is clean," I repeated. I checked the rest of the stomach and the duodenum, the adjacent part of the small intestine. "No ulcers anywhere else."

"I guess that's good," Penny said.

"Yes, that's very good. This means that he will probably recover pretty quickly. But we need to inject some epinephrine into the ulcer. Pass me the injection catheter."

Penny spoke from the corner.

"I've already flushed it with the epi so I'm ready to inject," she said. "I'll assist you whenever you're ready. I'm staying here so I don't crowd Mr. Hockey."

Hawkeye bit his lip but said nothing.

"Good. Let me get into position," I said.

Before I could inject, the oxygen alarm went off again.

"Stop! Wait! Don't do anything! I need to get his oxygen up! His oxygen's down to eighty-five percent. I just increased his oxygen to eight liters, I don't know what the heck is happening! He won't make it!"

Hawkeye re-adjusted the neck and suctioned furiously.

"I'm increasing the oxygen to ten liters," I said, worried.

Penny stepped forward again.

"Can I help? Can I hold his neck so you can suction?" she offered.

"No! I can handle it!"

"I just want to help you?"

"Do you think I can't handle it? Is that what you think?"

"No! Not at all."

"Then leave me alone! Go back to your corner!"

Penny looked at me, helplessly. I watched the monitor. The oxygen level climbed back quickly.

"Go back to your corner!" Hawkeye yelled. Penny hesitated.

The oxygen level returned to ninety-five percent. I sighed with relief.

"Okay, Penny. Come over here and help me with the injection."

Hawkeye was distressed.

"I don't know *what* the problem is, Doc. I swear, there's some kind of weird problem. He holds his oxygen level then it suddenly comes crashing down and I don't know why."

"Right now I need to focus on treating the ulcer."

"Yeah, sure. Go ahead. Only, I guess I'm sorry I haven't been much help keeping the oxygen level stable."

"Well, he's stable right now so let me hurry up and finish."

"Ten-four, Doc. I'm yanking his head so straight it's fixing to come right off! I've got his airway covered."

"Penny, inject half a cc of adrenaline now!"

Penny squeezed the syringe. I had inserted the needle at one corner of the ulcer. After the injection, the tissue swelled up and the puncture mark produced a wisp of red blood, which curled and floated in stomach acid. I watched the ulcer for a minute and nothing happened. I injected again thrice, encircling the ulcer with a circular blister of adrenaline. I slowly pulled the endoscope out.

"That was great! Are you going to do it again?" Penny asked.

"That's what the actress said to the bishop," Hawkeye sniggered.

Penny swung around and stopped short of punching him.

"Listen here, Hockey! That is so vulgar! You will *never* talk like that to me again, you hear? You cannot say that, okay? *Never!*" Penny was furious.

Hawkeye regarded her with cold amusement.

"You're really touchy," he observed. "How are you still married?"

"You just learn to behave, and maybe I won't kill you," Penny said. "Just maybe."

Penny and Hawkeye wheeled the patient out to the recovery area. I called Mr. Casteneda's wife and then informed Karl. I was completing my notes when Penny returned. She had a wry smile.

"Are you done with the paperwork, Doc?" she asked.

"Almost."

"No problem. He's waking up slowly."

"Any problems with his oxygen?"

"No," she said, and hesitated.

"What is it?" I asked.

"There is something I should tell you. It's kind of embarrassing."

I turned to look at her. She curled her hair with her fingers and scrunched her face.

"Don't tell Hockey. Doc, I was standing on the oxygen tubing," she admitted.

My jaw fell open.

"*What?*" I burst out.

"I was standing on the oxygen tubing. It was so long! I didn't realize it in the dark."

Penny shrugged with embarrassment. My mind reeled.

"So every time he sent you back to the corner, you ended up standing on the oxygen tubing!" I realized.

"Yes. And every time I came forward to help him, his oxygen went back up."

"Because you had stepped off the tubing!"

"Yes. I'm *so* sorry," Penny said. She stared at the floor.

I was still absorbing the news when Hawkeye returned.

"Penny, you need to come sit with your patient. I'm headed back to San Angelo. Doc, I need to apologize. I guess I was a bit cocky. I didn't do a good job. I'll try harder next time. I appreciate you being patient with me. I don't know why I couldn't keep that man's dang oxygen up!" he said, looking confused.

I glanced at Penny. She was silent.

"We all make mistakes," I said. "I'm glad the patient is doing well now. I do have a couple of cases tomorrow, starting at eight a.m."

"Okay! I'll be here, bright-eyed and bushy-tailed," Hawkeye said.

Hawkeye turned to Penny and spoke slowly and emphatically.

"Don't get in my face, nursy. I don't need your help to do my job, okay? I can do my job just fine. Just stay out of my way," he grumbled.

Penny shrugged. Hawkeye turned to leave.

"Next time, try to keep the patient's oxygen up, okay?" she taunted.

"Isn't that your job?"

Hawkeye scowled and turned to leave.

"Dr. Mathur really had a hard time because you couldn't keep the oxygen level up," she said, sharply. "You need to do better."

Hawkeye stiffened as he reached for the door. Penny was enjoying this.

"Don't let the door hit you where the Lord split you," she sang out.

Hawkeye swore and slammed the door.

CHAPTER 13
YOU'VE GOT TO LET GO

We drove down the winding road from Hotspur to Hord's Creek Lake. The girls were excited.

"This is so nice of Karl," Maya enthused.

"Yes, it is. He said I had been moping a lot since I had that complication and Dr. Wegener wrote that nasty review. Karl wanted to cheer me up."

"That's so nice of him to throw a party for you and call the entire office staff."

"Yes, it is. Apparently, he's done this a few times. He likes to call all the office staff along with their families out to the lake a couple of times a year."

"Well, he's making a special effort for you. Betty said that he's going to cook burgers and hot dogs and he's making some salmon patties for me."

"He's been unusually nice to me. It makes me nervous," I said.

"You're too nervous, really," Maya said. "You need to relax. Unwind a little. Let go!"

I sighed.

"What? You can't do it?" Maya asked.

"I'm a worrier," I said.

"You're strong-willed. Make yourself think of other things and stop thinking about the perforation. Stop worrying about the review. Remember, these things happen."

"I know. But I've never had one before."

"You've done so many procedures in London and Houston and now in Hotspur. So a complication was bound to happen eventually."

"I guess."

"Just how many colonoscopies have you done?"

"At least two thousand."

"Okay, So, your rate is one in two thousand. And she had risk factors. It wasn't entirely your fault."

I nodded but said nothing. We turned off the Winters Freeway and were waved through the turnstile.

"Karl paid the entrance fee for us," Maya said.

"Uh huh. Great," I muttered.

Maya watched my face and shook her head.

"You're wound up so tightly! You've got to unwind. This is going to be the perfect opportunity. I see a parking spot near site fourteen. Karl said to park there. We usually park near the restrooms, but Karl said to go past that area."

"Sure, whatever."

"Now stop moping! Enjoy the day and let go. It'll be good for you. Don't think about the perforation, don't worry about Dr. Wegener or the job in Austin or Abilene or moving out of Hotspur, or anything. Just enjoy the day, please! For everyone's sake," Maya pleaded.

I drove past our usual spot and parked near site fourteen. I helped Maya unstrap the girls from their car seats and took out a bag of towels from the trunk.

"Dad! Did you notice something about me?" Priya asked, bobbing her head from side to side.

I looked at her.

"I like your dress!" I ventured.

"No, look again!"

"You're wearing sunblock and you've got sunglasses, I see that."

"I got glasses too," Anjali announced.

"But what's new about me?" Priya asked again.

"You look so pretty!" I said.

"Dad! I got a *haircut!* How do you like my short hair?"

I flushed.

"Very nice. I like your haircut. You look better with short hair."

Priya beamed and picked up a towel.

"You need to unwind for your sake and for your family," Maya whispered as we walked to Karl's campsite.

Hord's Creek Lake is located west of Hotspur. It straddles Hord's Creek and was created by a long limestone dam, a tall embankment with control gates. A narrow road runs over it, lined with white metal fencing. We walked over it and joined Karl's party. Maya and I greeted Karl and his family, and the girls raced ahead. His campsite was at the junction of the embankment and the south shore. Karl and his family had strung lights, set up picnic tables and umbrellas, and had arranged chairs in clusters. Three large iceboxes with water and sodas lay open, and bags of potato chips, jars of mayonnaise and guacamole and bottles of ketchup and pickles graced every table. There was a wonderful smell of hamburgers frying and burning charcoal. Karl wore orange shorts and a Hawaiian T shirt and was busy talking to Tracy's husband, Trevor. I waved to them and flopped into a sagging deck chair.

I looked up. It was a magnificent cloudless blue sky. Gusts of wind blew fitfully and caressed the branches of the trees behind us and flattened the grass. Doves and blue jays and cottontails startled out of the trees and swooped in long arcs. They stalked the picnic tables, along with bumblebees and flies and hornets. Storks sat on the embankment fence, and ducks sunned themselves on the stones below. Clusters and straggling stems of marsh reeds and tall purple feathery grasses spotted the perimeter. Karl called out to Priya and Anjali and they came running back. They squealed with joy and hugged Karl. Karl took a step back and yanked off his sunglasses.

"You girls are getting awfully cute!" he declared. "Too dang cute!"

Priya and Anjali beamed. Karl clamped his shades back on.

"Want some hot dogs? Fries? Chips?"

They nodded vigorously.

"Get on back there! We got the whole office and their families here and my boys are feeding the lot. Get you some!"

The girls shot off.

"It's a beautiful day, Karl! Thanks for doing all this!" Maya said.

Karl embraced Maya and punched me on the shoulder.

"You know, Maya, we gotta get this dude to lighten up!" he said.

"That's exactly what I was telling him," Maya said. "He needs to lighten up."

I nodded wearily.

"I hear you, I hear you," I said. "This is already working. Karl, this place just looks so peaceful."

"Well, eat up and check out my jet skis!"

"What's a jet ski?"

Karl stopped flipping burgers. He pushed Trevor aside. He turned to me and lifted up his sunglasses.

"Are you telling me you don't know what a jet ski is?" he asked, incredulously.

"No," I admitted.

He looked at Trevor and they both shook their heads.

"I'm just shocked. Shocked! Shocked, I tell you. How did they give you American citizenship?"

"I don't have citizenship. I have a green card."

"How come you don't know what a jet ski is?" Maya looked at me in surprise.

"I don't know. I just haven't heard of it," I admitted.

Karl laughed.

"Your highness, you are a nerd. You are a turd. You live in an academic hole. No, *worse*. You don't live. You just work. You gotta *live!*"

I had nothing to say.

"Do you know how to live?" he asked me.

"Obviously not."

"You gotta camp out like this! Get you some hot dogs, burgers, fries and beer or cokes, then you get you a jet ski and you shoot across the lake and you yell and scream and you feel like a million bucks!"

"So a jet ski is like a water scooter?"

"Yeah. But it's more than that. Much more fun than that!"

"Does it ride like a bicycle?"

"Bicycle? Heck, no! It rides like a dang rocket!"

"How do you keep it upright?"

"It floats, Einstein. It floats. You just get on it like you was straddling a horse. Then you turn the handle and roll the dial and get you some power! And you have a good old time!"

"Great," I said, flatly.

Karl sat six burgers on six buns slathered with mayonnaise and laid two slices of thick cheese on the meat. He layered diced tomatoes and onions and topped it with sweet relish.

"I made you a veggie burger, your royal highness," he said.

"Thank you," I said.

"Bet you thought that I'd forget. No sir, I don't forget. I'm working on yours right now."

Karl handed me the tray with six burgers.

"These are regular burgers. Take these down to the gang. I got to cook one last round. Have the boys show you and Maya the jet skis and get on out there!"

I took the tray down to the waterfront. There was a smell of gently rotting vegetation and gasoline. Karl's older boys, Chad and Nate, were taking the children for rides on the two jet skis. Maya supervised them. We checked their life jackets.

"Boys, go slow! They're little, and they're not used to going fast," I warned.

"Yes, sir," they replied. "Father said to go slow and take it easy."

They pushed off the shore. They sped to the center of the lake and went round in loops, chasing each other. We heard the girls whoop and laugh and the boys yell at each other.

"Father sent these burgers and fries for you and Mrs. Mathur," a voice said.

I turned. It was Karl's youngest son, Jonah. He was tall and lanky, with brown hair and freckles. He had a wide smile.

"Thanks! I'm going to go talk to your mother," Maya said, and took one. She gazed at Jonah.

"Jonah! You have really changed! You've shot up!" she remarked.

"Yeah, I'm almost as tall as Chad. I'm as tall as Father, I reckon."

Maya went off to look for Betty, Karl's wife.

I took the plate from Jonah and looked for somewhere to sit down.

"How come you're not riding a jet ski?" I asked.

"I got a concussion so I'm not allowed on the water for a week."

"Were you playing football?"

"Nope. Soccer."

I was surprised. Jonah looked reluctant to discuss it further. I looked at the plate.

"What have you got for me?" I asked.

"Veggie burgers. Not as good as the veggie burgers I'm used to having," Jonah grinned.

I surveyed the plate. A bun with two veggie patties sat on a mound of French fries. The patties were covered with pesto and crowned with feta cheese crumbles and fried green peppers. I took a large bite. It was delicious.

"Better than this? Where have you been eating veggie burgers?" I asked.

"I work weekends at the motel. Mr. Patel and his wife, they're vegetarian. I'm friends with their son, Ram. She makes crazy good food! Love her cooking."

"What have you had?"

"Samosa and potato pancakes and sweet yogurt drinks and fried patties and lots of things."

"Isn't that food too hot for you?" I asked.

"Nah. I'm used to Mexican food. It's really spicy too."

I ate slowly, savoring the pesto and the fried peppers.

"Indian food is pretty spicy. Maybe more so."

"I can handle it. So do all the spices come from India?" Jonah asked.

"A lot of them do but peppers and potatoes originally came from South America, the New World."

"I thought green and red peppers came from India."

"They're grown there but they were brought there by Portuguese sailors and traders like Vasco da Gama. They were discovered in South America but wouldn't grow in Europe and sailors brought them to India. They grew really well there. Now they're essential for Indian food but they started off in South America."

"I didn't know that. Even potatoes came from South America?"

"Yes, even potatoes."

I munched a few fries. Jonah gathered a few flat rocks. Priya and Anjali were having a great time and Chad and Nate were careening the jet skis, making figures of eight and sending up walls of spray and foam, soaking each other.

"I heard of the potato famine in Ireland so I thought potatoes were always grown there," Jonah said.

"Actually, it's very interesting. The main crop in Europe used to be wheat. But wheat was temperamental and if there was bad weather or if the rains were poor or came at the wrong time, the crops failed."

"So there was always the threat of starvation?"

"Right. Europe was always on the brink of famine. Everyone was always worried about having enough to eat. And wheat didn't store well. It spoiled and got moldy."

Jonah reviewed his collection of flat stones.

"So how did potatoes help?" he asked.

"Potatoes were discovered in South America and brought to Europe where they did very well eventually. They were easier to grow. You just take a small piece of a potato with an eye, a dimple, and put it in the ground, and it grows into a full plant. The potatoes we eat are the swollen roots of the plant and each plant produced lots of potatoes. Potato plants didn't depend so much on the weather."

"What about storing them?"

"Potatoes store pretty well. Don't get moldy for a long time. Even if they sprout and start to grow they can still be eaten."

"So that fixed the famine problem?"

"Exactly. Then the Europeans could do other things like paint and sculpt and build great buildings. The Renaissance was due in part to the potato."

Jonah nodded. He started skimming stones on the water.

"The Renaissance was made possible by the humble potato," I repeated, grandly.

Jonah grunted and kept skimming stones.

"Hold off!" I said. "They're coming back."

The two jet skis roared back. They cut off power twenty feet away from the shore and came in slowly, bobbing gently. I waded out and retrieved Priya and Anjali.

"Can we do some more? Please?" Priya begged.

"More? Please!" Anjali chimed.

Karl walked up.

"Girls, get you something to eat. You got to eat while it's hot. Never miss a meal, okay? Remember that. Now your dad's going to go on the jet ski. Just watch him!" he boomed.

The girls went reluctantly to find Maya.

"Go ahead, your lordship, go ahead!" Karl insisted. I looked at the jet ski warily. It looked like a large white stag, rocking in the water

"Get your royal butt on that bad boy! Chad, give him your life jacket. Show him how to get on and how to accelerate."

With Chad's help I was able to mount the jet ski.

"Dr. Mathur, it's very simple. I'm going to slip this band around your wrist. In case you fall off the jet ski, this will turn it off so it will just wait for you to get back up. The accelerator is on the right side. You rotate it forwards and it goes forwards. You rotate it backwards, it slows down. Really simple."

I thanked him and turned it on. I headed towards the center of the lake, accelerating cautiously. I seemed to hit every wave, and my progress was slow and choppy. I remembered seeing Chad and Nate going smoothly. I realized that my speed was too low and I needed to accelerate.

I revved the engine. The jet ski leaped forward and I almost fell off. I shot ahead and cut through the water like a knife. I saw the other jet ski turn right so I banked and turned left and made a wide circle. I took another loop, and the jet ski bucked and shuddered as I hit more waves head on. The cold foam soaked me; it was exhilarating! I looped again and again, whooping with joy. I finally slowed down and headed back. I cut the power thirty feet from shore and covered the last stretch with an elegant drift.

"What the heck was that?" Karl asked. "A funeral? A funeral wake?"

I was stung.

"I went pretty fast!" I protested.

"Fast? Are you kidding? My grandma rides better than that!" Karl laughed.

"I was being careful," I explained.

"Careful? Careful not to have any fun? You're too slow! Here, let me show you how to do it."

I peeled off the band and shrugged off the life jacket. Karl slipped it on but didn't strap it closed. He jammed his sunglasses down and grabbed the handle. He leapt onto the seat in one fluid motion and gunned the engine. It roared, and the nose burst out of the water like a dolphin. Karl stood up and leaned in and the jet ski streaked away, nose well above the surface, the motor screaming, and an enormous plume of foam erupting from the propeller.

"Whoa! You *go*, Father!" Jonah marveled, pumping his fist.

Karl made tight turns and figures of eight and raced the jet ski like a motorcycle. He leaned to the left, and to the right, and leaned down so far it looked like he would hit the water. But he didn't. He straightened up and did it all again. And again. He leaned forwards, he leaned backwards. He suddenly flipped around and made a sharp loop while looking backwards. There was applause from the crowd. I joined in reluctantly.

"Father is *cool!*" Chad crowed.

Karl returned at breakneck speed. Ten feet from shore, he cut the power, leaned left, and made a ferocious U-turn. He soaked all of us and we heard him laugh. He made another loop and shot in again, making a sudden right turn to stop himself perfectly at the shoreline. His boys cheered. Karl jumped off and pointed to me.

"*That* is how you drive a jet ski, man! That is how you ski! *That* is how you live your life, man! *Wide ass open!*"

He hooted and whipped off the life jacket and tossed it to me. He peeled off his wet shirt and threw it to Nate.

"Man, that's living!" he exulted. He marched off, barefoot and shirtless, a rugged Adonis, completely disregarding his swooning audience. I watched with reluctant admiration. He leapt easily over a few boulders and disappeared.

I realized I had just seen a man who embodied everything I thought I was, or wanted to be, but wasn't.

* * *

Jonah brought me another burger.

"Your last one got wet when Father soaked us. Got you another."

I was still in thrall. I ate silently. Jonah squatted down and hunted for flat stones again. I watched him build up a pile. He inspected them and discarded a few. He stood up and started skimming the remaining stones.

"Father is getting the boat ready. We're going to go water-skiing. Have you ever done that before?" he asked.

"No."

"I didn't think so," he said.

I was stung. Jonah didn't notice.

"I don't think you'll like it. You didn't like the jet ski," he said.

"I did like the jet ski! It was just my first time ever, so I was just being careful," I explained.

"How come this was your first time?" Jonah asked.

"Well, all I did once I went to medical school was medicine. I didn't do anything else."

Jonah skimmed three stones in rapid succession.

"Are you a nerd?" he asked.

"Absolutely," I said. "A complete nerd."

Jonah grinned.

"That's okay if you really are a nerd," he said. "Or are you just saying that?"

"I'll prove it. You know, you stood up and skimmed some stones across the water, and you dropped some stones straight back on the ground."

"Some weren't good for skimming."

"I get that. But did you know that the stones that you dropped straight down to the ground and the stones you pitched out over the water, well, both hit the surface at the *same time*."

Jonah didn't even look up.

"No, they didn't. The stones that I threw over the water were in the air longer, then they turned down and hit the water. So they were in the air longer than the ones I just dropped."

"I thought so too, at first. Want to check it out?"

I puffed my chest, feeling important. Jonah shook his head. He wasn't convinced.

"You're wrong, Dr. Mathur. I'm really good at physics. I'm telling you, the ones I throw out over the water will hit the surface later than the ones I just drop to the ground," he insisted.

"Let's put it to the test," I said, and put my plate down.

We tried the experiment. Jonah skimmed a stone and I dropped one from the same height. It was close, and we couldn't be sure.

"I'm going to ask my science teacher tomorrow," Jonah declared. "I'll tell you what he says. He's really smart, he'll know."

It was getting late by the time we finally made it to the center of the lake. Karl was piloting the boat and gave orders.

"It's getting dark, so you boys will have to wait. We don't have enough time for everyone to ski. Let Maya try water skiing, she's a good swimmer."

Maya lowered herself into the water, wearing a bulky life jacket. She turned and moved into position. She strapped skis onto her feet and leaned back in the water. She grasped the bar that trailed from the back of the boat and leaned back until she was in the water to her shoulders, and the tips of the skis were sticking out if the water. She gave a thumbs up.

"So when I go, the rope will tighten up and pull you up out of the water," Karl bellowed over the idling motor. "Are you ready?"

"Yes, but go slow. This is my first time," Maya yelled back.

Karl nodded. He revved the engine. The boat jerked forwards and Maya cried out. She lost the bar and flopped in the water. Karl circled around and Nate tossed her the bar again.

"Okay, let's try this again," Karl said. He checked Maya, tested the rope, and accelerated. The rope whipped out of Maya's hands again. She settled herself and motioned for the rope a third time. The same thing happened again. I was surprised, because Maya is a strong swimmer and good at water sports.

Karl and Nate looked disappointed, but said nothing. Flushed with potential victory in the matter of gravity and skimming stones, I felt that I could use my superior command of physics to master water-skiing. It was up to me to save the family's honor.

"Let me try," I said, trying to sound confident.

"What? *You* water-ski? You, Mr. Royal Super Cautious Physician? *You?*" Karl wondered.

"Yes, me. Let me try. Try living, like you said."

Karl was surprised.

"Have you ever done this before?'

"No."

"Are you just trying to impress everyone?"

"No," I lied.

Karl stared at me in surprise, then shrugged.

"Then go for it, man!" he said.

I helped Maya out of the water and got in. I double-checked my life jacket and struggled to get my skis on. I leaned back in the water, bent my knees a little, and gripped the bar. I thought about my mastery of physics and imagined the optimal angle for my skis. Surely, all I had to do was keep my skis at forty-five degrees to the water surface and hold on very tightly to the bar. The forward acceleration of the boat would create an equal and opposite force from the water resistance against my skis. This force would pull me out of the water and I would slowly straighten up, keeping my center of gravity behind my shoulders at all times. Maya's mistake, I reasoned, was that she kept letting go of the bar. Therefore, the boat's momentum was not being transmitted to her. *I* would not let go. I pointed my skis out at what I thought was a perfect angle, bent my knees slightly more, and gave an enthusiastic thumbs up.

Suddenly, the world went dark and I was deep underwater. I was at the bottom of the lake. It was grey and cold and silent, with strands of light and a great pressure crushed my chest. I desperately wanted to open my mouth and scream and breathe but forced myself not to do that. I clamped my jaws together. I looked up and arched back, still grasping the bar for dear life. I went rigid, my face and neck engorged and throbbed violently and I fought the mounting urge to open my mouth and inhale. Seconds went by. I remained frozen and couldn't think.

The rope tightened and I was wrenched up to the surface. My face shot out of the water, but I was too scared to take a breath. I waited to make sure that my mouth was not surrounded by water and then took a quick gasp. My airway was so tight that I could only manage a few whistling breaths. Slowly, the airway spasms subsided. I sucked the air in deeply, curling and straightening with the effort. I heard Maya and Karl in the boat calling my name. They turned back and threw me another rope. I grabbed it and was pulled into the boat. Maya looked terrified. Karl was beside himself.

"What is wrong with you, man?" he stormed. "What is *wrong* with you? You're supposed to let go quickly if you don't ride up! Don't you *ever* know when to let go?"

I had no air to spare for words. I heard Karl loud and clear.

"Damn internists! They just hang on!" he howled.

That's it, that's exactly my problem, I thought. *I don't know when to let go.*

CHAPTER 14
THE MERCHANT OF VENICE

We drove back home silently until Priya spoke.

"So Daddy could have *died?*" she asked, incredulously.

Maya hesitated.

Priya reared up, grabbed the back of my seat, and asked again.

"Is that right? Daddy almost *died* in the water?"

Maya nodded.

"That's so scary!" Priya declared. "What would we do if Daddy died?"

Anjali looked glum and upset.

"It was a mistake. Don't worry, everything's fine," I reassured them.

"You almost *died*, Dad!" Priya cried.

We were shaken and silent. I was shocked by what had just happened.

"Everything's fine. I'm fine, don't worry," I repeated.

"I scared," Anjali said.

"I'm fine, really. Everything is okay. Really, it is. Look at me."

"Really?" Anjali asked.

"Really," I said, firmly.

Priya and Anjali pondered for a few minutes.

"Everything's okay?" Priya wondered.

"Yes, yes," I insisted. "Everything's back to normal."

"I scared," Anjali repeated.

"There's nothing to be scared about. Everything's okay now," I promised.

"I'm scared too," Priya whimpered. I glanced back at them. They looked close to tears.

"You can have a nice hot bath and Mom and I will sit in your room until you go to sleep," I said.

That reassured them.

"So will you tell us a story?" Priya asked. Anjali nodded vigorously.

Maya looked out the window and shook her head.

"Sure. What kind of story?" I smiled.

"A long story."

"An Akbar and Birbal story?"

"No, no. We've heard them all, Dad."

"But you like them so much!"

"How about one little Akbar and Birbal story and then one new long story?" Priya pleaded.

Maya looked at me.

"Are you up to it? Maybe just end the day now?" she wondered. "Don't forget, you have to finish an art project with Anjali."

"I'm still charged up. I think sitting down in their room with the lights turned out and telling them a story will help calm me down. I just don't feel like doing an art project right now."

An hour later, everyone had bathed and changed into pajamas. The lights had been turned off and the girls were in bed. Maya and I sat on the floor of the girls' bedroom in the darkness.

"Tell a long story!" Priya insisted.

"Tell Akbar Birbal," Anjali requested.

"Okay, one Akbar and Birbal story first. Once upon a time, hundreds of years ago, there was a great king in India. Do you remember what his name was?"

"Akbar!" the girls chorused.

"Correct! And who was Birbal?"

"His best friend!"

"Actually, he was Akbar's prime minister. That means, he was the person who advised the king about what to do."

"Okay, okay."

"So, one day it turned out that Birbal had made a big mistake. He had messed something up and it had cost Akbar a lot of money to fix the problem. So Akbar decided that Birbal should pay a fine."

"What's a fine?"

"That's when you have to give some of your own money to someone else as a punishment."

"How much money?"

"Hold on. So Birbal said to Akbar, oh great King Akbar, you can see that I made a mistake and I agree to pay a fine. But I ask you a favor. Let me choose three judges and explain my mistake. Then let them decide how much money I should pay as a fine."

"Why didn't he just pay the fine, Dad?"

"He knew that the King was upset and would make him pay a lot of money."

"But the other three people could have made him pay even more!"

"This is where Birbal was clever. He selected three poor people as the judges!"

"Then what happened?"

"He brought three very poor people into the court in front of the King. He explained what he had done wrong. The three poor people asked Birbal how much damage he had caused."

"So then they could fine him?"

"Yes. Birbal told them that he had caused a lot of damage. Then he asked them to fine him a lot of money."

"He *told* them to fine him a lot of money? Why?"

"He said that he was sorry for causing the damage."

"How much did they want him to pay?"

"Well, the three men were very poor. They had never seen much money. So they said, okay, let's fine Birbal five rupees or ten rupees."

"Only five or ten rupees? That's not much money!" Priya protested.

"Yes, but to poor people it was a lot of money. So one of the poor people fined Birbal five rupees, another one ten rupees and the third one fifteen rupees, because, *for them*, that was a lot of money."

"So Birbal didn't have to pay a lot of money!"

"Right! Birbal knew that if the rich King had fined him, he would have asked for a lot of money, maybe thousands of rupees. But for poor people, even five or ten or fifteen rupees seemed like a lot of money."

"So Birbal got away without having to pay a lot of money!"

"Exactly! He knew that everyone sees things from their own background. A rich man thinks nothing of thousands of rupees and a poor man thinks that ten rupees is a lot of money. So the clever Birbal got a very small fine because he asked poor people to judge him and fine him what *they* thought was a lot of money."

"Birbal was very clever," Priya nodded.

"Yes, he was. Now, are you up for another story or are you too sleepy?"

"Yes, yes! Ready!" Priya cried.

"Yes! Story!" Anjali whooped.

Maya interrupted.

"This is not a good idea. You're tired and you should sleep," she repeated.

"I've got a good story for them. The Merchant of Venice."

"The Shakespeare story? That's much too long."

"They wanted a long story. Why not this one? I think they'll like it."

"We want the long story!" Priya insisted.

"Long story! Long story!" Anjali cried.

Maya sighed.

"Well, they don't sound sleepy. Go ahead," she said.

"Okay, let's start. A long time ago, in Italy, there was a city called Venice. Venice was right on the edge of the sea, and so many people had big boats and used them to send nice things from Italy to other countries and bring back other nice things from those places. These people were called merchants, and some of them became very rich."

"They became rich by sending things to other countries?"

"Yes. They would sell nice Italian things like wine and cheese and paintings for a lot of money in far-away countries and bring back things from those countries that the Italians wanted, and they made a lot of money. So Venice became a very rich city. And there lived in Venice, a very nice and rich merchant called Antonio."

"Everyone liked Antonio?" Priya asked.

"Yes. Everyone liked him because he was happy and cheerful and also because he would lend money without interest."

"What's interest?"

"Well, when you lend someone your money, lets say, a hundred dollars, then you should get your money back, a hundred dollars, after some time, say, a month. But you could also say, well, I'm going to give you a hundred dollars and I want you to give me back one hundred and ten dollars in one month."

"Why should you get more?"

"Because you didn't get to keep your money and spend it and you're not enjoying your money. Also, if you lend money to a lot of people, some of them might not pay you back, so you need to get a little extra back from the others just in case."

"Okay. So that extra money is the interest?"

"Exactly. The extra money you want back is the interest. So Antonio was very nice and he didn't charge any interest. But there was another person in Venice who had a lot of money and his name was Shylock. Shylock did charge money when he gave someone a loan."

"Did people like Shylock?

"No, they didn't like Shylock. He charged interest and Antonio didn't, and Antonio even made fun of Shylock in front of everyone."

"Antonio is nice, like Dr. Becker," Priya decided.

"Well, yes, Dr. Becker is very nice and popular."

"And he lets everyone borrow his things for free, like his boats and his jets."

"Jet skis. Yes, he lets everyone borrow for free."

"He makes fun of you, so you're like Shylock."

Maya laughed.

"Hold on! If I had things to lend, I would lend them for free," I protested.

"But he does make fun of you, and you don't like it," Priya persisted.

"Well, in this story, Shylock is the bad guy, and I don't want to be the bad guy."

"Okay, then. Go on."

"So Antonio, the good merchant, and Shylock, the bad merchant, lived in Venice. Shylock didn't like Antonio because Antonio was always making fun of him and so he wanted to get his revenge."

"Do you want to get your revenge on Dr. Becker?"

"Why would I want to get revenge on Dr. Becker?" I asked.

"Because he almost drowned you."

"No, don't be silly. He didn't try to drown me. That was my mistake. I don't know how to ski and I shouldn't have tried it."

"So you're not mad at him?"

"No. Now listen to the story. Antonio had a very good friend called Bassanio. Bassanio was in love with a lady called Portia."

"Was she beautiful?"

"Yes."

"Did she have long hair?"

"Yes."

"Long black hair?"

"Yes. No, blonde. I think she had blonde hair."

"I blond. I born in Texas, I *blond*," Anjali declared.

"No, you have brown hair," Priya corrected.

"I *going* to be blond," Anjali insisted. "Because I Texan."

"So Antonio's friend Bassanio loved Portia and wanted to marry her. But he needed a lot of money to impress her. Bassanio didn't have the money so he asked Antonio. Normally, Antionio had plenty of money but on that day he didn't have any."

"Why?" Priya asked.

"Because his ships were all away in different places and hadn't returned. He had spent all his money buying things to send in his ships and so he didn't have any money left. So he went and asked Shylock for the money."

"But Shylock didn't like Antonio!"

"Right! That was a big mistake. Now Shylock thought, here's a chance for me to get even with Antonio. So he pretended to be nice and said to Antonio, sure, I'll lend you the money."

"And charge a lot of interest!" Priya guessed.

"No. He said, I won't charge any interest at all. But, just for fun, if you can't return the money in exactly two weeks, then as punishment, I want a pound of your flesh."

"What? A *pound* of Antonio's *flesh*?" Priya was aghast. "You mean, cut off a piece of his body?"

"Yes. Shylock said it was just a joke. He said, just for fun, if you don't return the money in two weeks then I will cut off a part of your body with a sharp knife!"

"That's horrible! That's not a joke. He wanted to cut off a piece of Antonio!" Priya howled. Anjali whimpered and shook her head in disapproval.

"He could have cut his head or his hand or his heart!" Priya went on, shocked.

"Bad! Bad!" Anjali cried.

"Well, Antonio thought that it was all a joke and that he would soon have the money, so he agreed. Antonio and Shylock signed a paper and Shylock gave Antonio the money, three thousand ducats. And Antonio gave the money to Bessanio."

"Bessanio should have told Antonio not to do it!" Priya said.

"Yes, he told Antonio not to make that deal with Shylock, but Antonio took the money and gave it to Bessanio. Bessanio and his servant Gratiano went to see the beautiful lady Portia."

"How did that go?" Priya asked.

"Bessanio impressed Portia with his nice clothes and his nice personality. And his servant, Gratiano, impressed Nerissa."

"Wait, wait. Now who are these new persons?"

"Gratiano was Bessanio's servant, and Nerissa was Portia's maid."

"Can we call them some thing easier?"

"Okay. What would you like?"

"Just make it simpler."

"Okay. The main people are the good guy Antonio, his friend, Bessanio, the bad guy, Shylock, and the beautiful lady, Portia."

"Okay. But why didn't Antonio have a girlfriend?"

"Don't know. It wasn't in this story. Maybe in another story. But Bessanio's servant was Gratiano and we can call him Graz and Portia's maid was Nerissa and we can call her Neri."

"Okay. Did Mrs. Potion agree to marry him?"

"Yes, she did. In fact, Lady Portia agreed to marry Bessanio, and her maid Neri agreed to marry Bessanio's servant, Graz!"

"Because they were rich?"

"Bessanio told her that he wasn't really very rich, and that he had borrowed the money from his friend, Antonio. Portia gave Bessanio a ring as a present and they made preparations for a big wedding. Her maid, Neri, gave Graz a ring, too."

"But what happened to Antonio?"

"Three weeks went by and then Bessanio got a message from Antonio. It was very bad news. Antonio's ships had not returned and so he didn't have any money to give to Shylock. The two weeks had gone by and now Shylock was insisting on cutting off a piece of Antonio. They were sure that Shylock was going to cut out Antonio's heart so that he could kill him!"

"What? He was so mean!" Priya cried out.

"So mean!" Anjali echoed.

The phone rang in the kitchen. Maya got up, and I pulled her down.

"It's probably for me, at this time of night," I sighed.

"We want to hear the story!" Priya complained.

"Dad will be right back," Maya said, soothingly. "This is why I don't like him starting these long stories late at night."

* * *

"Hello! This is Dr. Mathur," I answered.

"Yo, Einstein!" Karl bellowed.

"Karl? What's the matter?"

"Just checking on you. You swallowed half the lake, you know. Probably got flesh-eating ameba and other junk by now. You still alive?"

"Yes."

"Not dead?"

"No."

"So you're going to come to work Monday?"

"Yes."

"Unless you come down with meningitis or flesh-eating bacteria or something?"

"Right. Karl, what's up?"

"My dad's best friend has some bleeding going on. Bleeding from the rear end. He's been to see the specialists in Abilene and Dallas and he isn't getting any better. Still bleeding like a stuck pig. Will you see him Monday?"

"Sure, man. Bye!"

"You sound pissed off."

"No, I'm not."

"You need to unwind, man. You're wound tighter than a two-year clock."

"I appreciate your concern."

"Oh, so touchy! Still mad about your skiing disaster? Thought you were going to look like James damn Bond, zipping past all the pretty ladies, and sipping a martini?"

"I miscalculated, okay?"

"I heard you were spouting physics, Einstein. Did you think that you were going to use physics to water-ski?"

"I just thought I could be logical and position my center of gravity better than Maya. I read about it once."

"Read about it? That's ridiculous! A little learning is a dangerous thing," Karl said, drily.

"Thank you, Karl."

"Hey, man, you're welcome. See you Monday!"

I hung up and returned to the girls' bedroom.

* * *

"Finish the story, Dad!"

"Where were we?"

"The bad man was going to kill the good man because the good man couldn't return the money."

"Right. Antonio, the good man, didn't have the money, so Shylock, the bad man, was going to cut off a piece of Antonio's body."

"He could cut the flesh off from somewhere else like the legs," Priya suggested helpfully. Anjali nodded vigorously in support.

"He could have, yes. But Shylock wanted to get rid of Antonio so he was preparing to cut Antonio's heart out and that way he could kill Antonio and no one could say anything to him because Antonio had agreed to it."

"But that's not fair! You can't just kill someone!" Priya cried.

"I know, Priya, but those times were different. And poor Antonio had signed the contract that said that Shylock could take a pound of his flesh. The contract didn't say from where, so Shylock was free to cut off a pound of flesh from anywhere."

"How much is a pound?"

"Remember that bag of flour we used for Mom's cake?"

"The big white bag of flour? It was heavy!"

"That's a pound. So Shylock was going to cut a pound of flesh away from Antonio and Antonio knew and everyone knew that Shylock was going to kill Antonio in front of everyone, and there was nothing anyone could do about it."

"What is flesh?" Anjali asked.

I smiled.

"Flesh is skin and muscle."

"Okay."

"So Bessanio was very upset. He told Portia what had happened and that he had to go to see Antonio."

"He's *got* to save Antonio!" Priya cried.

"Well, he didn't really have any ideas but did take three times the money that Antonio owed. He offered Shylock three times the money if he would leave Antonio alone."

"What did Shylock say?"

"Shylock said no. Shylock didn't want the money. He just wanted to kill Antonio."

"Dad, if you were Shylock, would you take the money?" Priya asked earnestly.

"I wouldn't have ever asked for a pound of flesh, Priya! What makes you think I would be like that?"

"I'm just asking, Dad. Just suppose if Dr. Becker were Antonio and you were Shylock, just suppose, just suppose, then would you take the money or kill Antonio?"

"I would definitely not kill Antonio. I would not take the money, either," I said, vehemently.

"I think you should take the money," Priya said. "After all, Dr. Becker was mean to you. He made fun of you in front of everyone."

"That's his style. But he's really a good man and I know it. He has helped me out many times. So I would never want to hurt him."

Priya was reassured. Maya was amused and I could make out that she was smirking.

"Okay, good. Go on, Dad."

I was bothered by the comparison.

"Now Portia came up with a plan. She talked to a clever lawyer and told him the whole story. The clever lawyer told her what to do. He told her to dress like a man and pretend to be a lawyer."

"Why did she have to dress like a man?"

"Because in those days only men could be lawyers."

"That's not fair!" Priya and Anjali chorused indignantly.

"It was not fair," I conceded. "But that's how life was, a long time ago."

"Can girls be lawyers now?"

"Absolutely! They can be anything they want."

"Can they drive ships and planes?"

"Yes. They can even be astronauts, which means they can fly rockets."

The girls nodded and settled down.

"So Portia pretended to be a man and dressed up as a lawyer and went to Venice. She had a letter from the real lawyer, saying that she was a lawyer, and that she should be allowed to take part in the case and help Antonio."

"Did they let her?"

"Yes. The judge in charge said Portia could defend Antonio. Remember, Portia was disguised as a man and even Bessanio did not recognize her. Bessanio was the man who was going to marry her."

"What about the maid, Neri?"

"She also dressed up as a man and pretended to be an assistant lawyer."

"Did the judge also want Antonio to die?"

"No, only Shylock wanted Antonio to die. Everyone else loved Antonio."

"Go on, Dad! You're taking too long."

"I thought you wanted a long story," I teased.

"Dad, you're taking too long! Did the good man die? Tell us what happened!"

"All right. So the clever Portia spoke to Shylock in front of everyone and asked Shylock to take the money, a lot more money, nine thousand ducats instead of three thousand, but Shylock said no. Then Portia asked him to show mercy."

"What mercy?" Anjali asked, yawning, her voice drowsy.

"Mercy means forgiving people for their mistakes."

"Is that good?" Priya wondered.

"Mercy is a very good thing. Mercy means to forgive people. Everyone makes mistakes, and we need to forgive people when they make a mistake and they didn't mean to be bad. Portia told Shylock that when you forgive people, you get a blessing from God as well as the person you're being nice to, so you get two blessings for every act of mercy."

"Did Shylock forgive Antonio?"

"No. He just sat in a corner, sharpening his knife. He was looking forward to cutting open poor Antonio and killing him in front of everyone."

"So Antonio died?" Priya asked, agitated.

"This is the best part. Portia told Shylock that he should go ahead and cut off a pound of flesh from any part of Antonio because the contract clearly said so."

"What? *No!* That's not fair! It's not fair!" Priya protested.

"Listen to what she *also* said. Portia also said three very clever things. The first thing she said was, you can have a pound of flesh but you can't have any of his blood. So Shylock was totally confused! How could he cut off a pound of flesh without spilling any blood? That was impossible. You can't cut flesh without causing bleeding. And the contract did not say anything about taking Antonio's blood! So he couldn't cut Antonio."

"Yay! That's so clever!"

"Then she said another clever thing. She said, you can have exactly one pound and not a bit more. If you take more than one pound exactly, you will be guilty of murder! But there was no way Shylock could be so exact. So Shylock was trapped again!"

Priya clapped with delight. Anjali nodded.

"And then Shylock realized that he couldn't win. He couldn't cut flesh without spilling blood, and there was no mention of blood in the contract. Also, there was no way he could be sure of cutting out exactly one pound, no more, so he was in double trouble! So he agreed to take the money."

"So they gave him the money? And he went away?"

"No. Portia had one last clever thing to say. She said, because you were plotting to hurt a citizen of Venice, the law says we can take away all your money and give half to Antonio and the other half to the government and you will have no money at all."

"So Antonio got rich again!"

"Antonio was a good man and he pardoned Shylock. He told Shylock to be kind to everyone in the future and to never be cruel, and Shylock agreed. And everyone was so happy!"

"Did they figure out it was Portia?"

"No, not right away. Bessanio and Graz were so grateful to the lawyer, who was really Portia, that they offered anything in reward. Portia and Neri decided to test them. As a reward, Portia asked Bessanio for the ring that she herself had just given him. And Portia's maid, Neri, who was also dressed as a man and was pretending to be an assistant lawyer, asked Bessanio's servant, Graz, for his ring too."

"The one that she had given him?"

"Yes."

"So did the boys give up the rings?"

"Yes. They didn't want to, but they felt that the lawyers had done such an amazing job that they had to give them the rings."

"That wasn't nice!" Anjali declared.

"Well, Bessanio and Graz were so grateful that they gave up the rings."

"They should not have given up their rings," Priya decided.

"Well, they felt that the lawyers had just saved Antonio's life. So they really wanted to thank them."

"Even then. They should have found some other way."

"Finally, when Bessanio and Graz went back to Portia and Neri, they took Antonio with them. Portia and Neri had changed back and were dressed as fine ladies. They pretended to be very angry that the rings were gone."

"But they had them, right?"

"Right, because they themselves were the lawyers who had helped save Antonio. So they just pretended to be angry. Then they gave Bassanio and Graz the rings back."

"That's how the boys figured out the lawyers were actually the two girls!" Priya said, triumphantly.

"Exactly! And Graz's ring had special words written on it."

"What did it say?"

"It said, Love me ever, leave me never."

"That's so sweet," Priya sighed.

"Sweet, so sweet," Anjali mumbled, sleepily.

"Now we're all going to be quiet and go to sleep," Maya said, firmly.

We sat in the darkness for another ten minutes until there was unbroken silence.

As we tiptoed out, Maya grasped my wrist.

"*Love me ever, leave me never.* That's the inscription on the bracelet you gave me," she whispered.

"Yes," I admitted.

"I thought you came up with it yourself. But it wasn't original!" Maya hissed in mock anger.

I grinned.

"You're right. I Bard it," I said.

CHAPTER 15

THE MAN WHO KEPT ON BLEEDING

It was Monday morning. I was in the clinic office, talking to Tracy.

"You really scared us, Dr. Mathur. We panicked when you went under the water and didn't come up."

"It was the scariest moment of my life," I admitted.

"You know, there are a lot of grasses and stuff at the bottom. Your feet could have gotten caught in them."

"I didn't realize that."

"Getting your feet out of the skis would have been really difficult, especially if you had panicked. Good thing you held on to the rope!" Tracy said.

I shuddered as I recalled the event.

"I was very lucky," I said.

The door was kicked open and Karl sauntered in. He wore a baseball cap, a black T-shirt that said *Semper Fi*, denim jeans and a fresh white coat. He grinned and pointed at me.

"Yo, Einstein!" Karl whooped.

I looked at Karl. I was still thinking of my underwater adventure.

"Einstein! I'm talking to you!" Karl bellowed.

"What?"

"I got that patient for you, man with bleeding, remember, I told you?"

"Yes."

"Friend of my dad. Herschel. Herschel Dunn. Lives out in the country. I think you did some kind of crazy home visit on him when you had your ass kicked out of the hospital last year."

That irritated me.

"I was never kicked out of the hospital! My hospital privileges were on hold, that's all."

"Why they were on hold, Einstein?" Karl boomed.

I sighed. Karl knew all the details.

"I think everyone here knows all the details."

"Enlighten us, Majesty."

"There was a patient who had a cardiac arrest. I was helping resuscitate him. He had a low potassium level, so I gave him an IV bolus of potassium. There was a locum here, Dr. Ehrlich, from Dallas. He didn't think the patient needed potassium. I gave it against his orders anyway. We lost the patient a few minutes later. Dr. Ehrlich was very angry and suspended me from the staff while there was an investigation."

Karl snorted.

"Suspended. Fired. Same difference."

"There was an inquiry and they backed me up completely. In fact, the investigator was an ICU nurse who said we could press charges against Dr. Ehrlich for *not* giving the potassium."

"The patient died anyway, right, Einstein?"

"Forget it. You want me to see Herschel Dunn? I remember Herschel from that home visit. What's going on?"

"He's been bleeding for weeks. He's got this drip, drip, drip of blood. It's all over his shorts and even on his pants! He's wearing diapers now and has to change them three or four times a day."

"What's his hemoglobin?"

"Seven point one."

I whistled. The office manager, Tracy, looked up.

"Is that bad?" she asked.

"Normal's twelve to fourteen, so he's lost almost half his blood," Karl muttered.

"Did he have a blood transfusion?"

"He's getting one right now. I also gave him a colon cleanout. In case your highness wants to do a colonoscopy."

I sat up straight.

"Is it bright red blood or black tarry stuff?" I asked.

"It's bright red. It's liquid, constantly dripping out his rear end."

"So it's likely to be coming from the lower left colon or rectum. If it were coming from higher up, it would turn black by the time it came out," I said.

"Everyone knows that. I'm almost done giving him two units of packed red cells. Want to do the colonoscopy? See what's bleeding?"

"Sure. Great idea."

Karl hesitated.

"Full disclosure: I panicked when I saw him bleeding a couple weeks ago and I sent him over to Wegener in Abilene."

I stiffened. Karl grinned.

"You have a long history with Wegener, don't you?"

"You know I do," I snapped.

"Heard he wouldn't even talk to you. Jacked with you. Gave you the cold shoulder," Karl chuckled.

I nodded. The memory was painful.

"Basically kicked your ass."

"Thanks, Karl."

"But Herschel's still bleeding. Wegener couldn't fix him."

"What did Wegener do for Herschel?" I asked. "Let me guess. Upper endoscopy and colonoscopy?"

"Wegener stuck a scope into Herschel's mouth and up his backside. Never did get an official report. Wife said the stomach was fine but he had radiation damage somewhere, she didn't know where. Put old Herschel on iron tablets and steroids and sent him home."

I thought for a minute.

"Hang on. Didn't Herschel have prostate cancer about five or six years ago?"

"Yes. How'd you remember that?"

"For a man like Herschel to have rectal bleeding from radiation, the most likely cause is prior radiation therapy for prostate cancer. Radiation to the prostate may cause the rectal lining to get damaged and start bleeding. It would cause that regular drip of bright red blood. That diagnosis explains the whole story."

"But why would Wegener give Herschel steroids for that?"

"He probably prescribed steroid enemas, not tablets. Steroid enemas can be used to treat radiation damage."

Karl nodded.

"So you just squirt the stuff up your rear end?" Karl asked.

"Yep."

"Every day?"

"Every night."

"Crap! For how long?"

"Two or three weeks. It's not so bad."

Karl shook his head ferociously.

"Far as I'm concerned, that's an outie. Stuff comes out of there. Nothing goes in," Karl huffed.

"Well, if you're bleeding there, that's where the medicine should go."

"I don't like it. Anyway, I got old Herschel lined up to do a colonoscopy by me, but then I figured, hey, you're the *specialist*. Why not get *you* to do the scope and check out his rear end?"

I shrugged

"I'll be glad to do it. I have a hunch I'm right about the radiation damage. I'm going to have the pharmacy prepare a special solution that should stop his bleeding."

"You're sure that's causing the bleeding?" Karl asked, surprised

"Yes. I'm pretty sure he has radiation damage in the rectum."

"Without even seeing the patient? You're that sure of your diagnosis?"

"Yes, based on what you've told me. Making the diagnosis is straightforward, but treating it is difficult. Any other history?"

"He's an eighty year old black male, married, lives out in the country.

Had a triple bypass ten years ago, now he's got atrial fibrillation but no angina. Got a pacemaker. He has diabetes but controls it with diet alone."

"If he has atrial fibrillation he's probably on warfarin," I said. "Warfarin is a blood thinner and will aggravate his bleeding."

"Makes sense."

"Does he have a plain pacemaker or a pacemaker-defibrillator?" I asked.

Karl looked exasperated.

"What do you mean?"

"Is his pacemaker just a pacemaker or is it also a defibrillator?"

"Don't know. Why is that important?"

"Because if his heart is really weak and he's got serious heart failure, typically they put in a pacemaker-defibrillator. If there's a rhythm problem but no heart failure you get a plain pacemaker and no defibrillator. So it helps to know which one he has; it tells you a lot about his heart condition."

Karl was intrigued.

"Why put in a defibrillator if there's a weak heart?" he asked.

"When the heart is weak, let's say congestive heart failure with an ejection fraction less than thirty-five percent, then he's at high risk of fatal heart rhythms like ventricular tachycardia and fibrillation."

"Is ventricular tachycardia and fibrillation the same thing as v-tach and v-fib?" Tracy asked.

Karl nodded thoughtfully.

"Yeah, Trace, it is. With v tach and v fib, the heart rhythm becomes so irregular it's like the heart just stopped working. I've actually seen that happen. I was at a hospital New Year's party. Smack in the middle of it, a doctor just keeled over and dropped dead! Turned out, he had severe heart failure and was on a transplant list. Just had an attack of v tach. We couldn't save him. Died right there in front of his wife and about fifteen other doctors," Karl recalled. Tracy gasped.

"Exactly. So if he has a pacemaker that's also a defibrillator, then he's got pretty bad heart failure. If he has a pacemaker without a defibrillator then his heart's not so bad."

"I'm pretty sure it's only a pacemaker, but I'll ask again. "

"Thanks, but I can ask him when I see him," I offered.

"There you go, all slimy and superior again. Just because you know some stuff about pacemakers. Tell me something else, Sherlock! Look at me and tell me something else."

I looked at his shirt and baseball cap.

"You're wearing a Semper Fi T-shirt and I know you weren't in the Marines. The only one in your family whose shirt would fit you is your dad, so I'm guessing your dad was a Marine. And you're an Astros fan."

Karl smiled happily.

"Wrong on both. Got this T-shirt from a friend and this hat at a church sale."

I was deflated.

"Wrong on both!" Karl crowed.

"Okay," I shrugged.

"So will you do it?" Karl asked.

"Do the colonoscopy?"

"Yes, Einstein, the colonoscopy."

"Sure. Thanks for asking me."

Karl nodded. He stood up and ambled towards a clinic room.

"Where is Herschel?" I asked.

"He's in the old OR. The new OR had a water leak. We're waiting on Hawkeye."

I hurried over. The old Operating Room was in a part of the hospital that was mainly used for storage. It was a windowless room, fifteen feet by twenty feet, with white tile on the walls and floor and fluorescent tubes and a surgical lamp array hanging from the ceiling. The room smelled of phenol and iodine. The room was too bright and I turned off the overhead surgical lamps as I entered.

Herschel was lying on a narrow hospital bed. Penny had just completed the blood transfusion and was discarding the tubing. She connected a bag of saline to the same IV port.

Herschel was a thin, clean-shaven black man, with a halo of cropped white hair. He sat up on one elbow as I entered and extended his other hand. He grinned widely.

"By golly, is that you? Dr. San-dip? Is that you?"

"Hello Herschel! So good to see you again."

"I'm tickled pink, Dr. San-dip! You remember me?" he said, laughing at the memory.

"Of course I do! I saw you in your home last year when you had pneumonia. You refused to come to the hospital!"

Herschel laughed.

"Yeah, I can be stubborn as a mule, I can. Old Bill Hennessy, he drug you out of the hospital to come see me. You fixed me right up! As you can see, I made it, Doctor San-dip!"

"I'm delighted! You never came for follow up but Bill told me you were better. I keep meeting Bill in the Shopping Basket."

"That Bill, he's a good guy. Like a brother to me. You know, his daddy taught me and Bill and my kid brother, Clarence, how to play baseball. He was a good man, Bill's dad, he was. You know, when he was young, Old Man Hennessy, he was selected by the Boston Red Sox, did you know that?"

"Yes, Bill mentioned it. Why didn't he join?"

"Bill's dad enlisted and joined the army instead. Said it was his duty to protect his country. It was the Second World War. When he came back they didn't want him no more. So he and his wife came down to Texas where she owned land."

"Around Hotspur?"

"Uh-huh. But when they first moved here they bought them a house on Westmoreland Street, in the Black part of town."

"There was a *Black* part of town? In tiny Hotspur?"

"Oh, yeah. It was pretty bold of them. Then they built a ranch house and moved there couple three years later. Been ranching ever since."

"I'm surprised that a small town like Hotspur had a Black part of town."

"Sure did. Still does. Black grocery store, Black church, Black undertaker. Still does."

I pulled up a metal stool and sat down as I took this in. I forced myself to focus.

"What's happening to you now?" I asked.

Herschel sighed and laid down.

"It's crazy, Dr. San-dip. I just keep on bleeding. I'm passing a little bit of blood every time I go to the bathroom."

"Every time you pass urine also?"

"No, I mean every time I do number two. And I go three, sometimes four times a day."

"How much blood comes out? A few drops or a big gush or blood clots?"

"Like someone painted red all over my BM."

"Is it mixed in with your BM?"

"No. It's on top and separate. But there's an awful lot of it sometimes."

"I'm looking at your chart. I see your hemoglobin was down to just under seven grams percent. Seven grams! That's really low. That's the level we transfuse blood."

Herschel waved his hands in protest.

"No more blood! No more blood! I don't want no AIDS or nothing! I got this blood 'cause Dr. Karl said I was fixing to have a stroke or heart attack."

"He's right."

"I said, just give me what I got to have so I don't get a stroke or something. No more than that, I don't want to get AIDS!"

"Blood is always checked for the AIDS virus but there could be other viruses that we don't know about. Your blood level is pretty low, sir, you're right on the borderline of needing more blood than just two units."

"No. No more blood. I'm scared. What else can we do?"

"We can give you iron by mouth or iron by vein instead."

"I'm taking an iron pill every day."

"That may not be enough. You should increase it to twice daily, and take it with orange juice or vitamin C. That will increase the absorption."

"I can do that."

"Have you checked your B12 level?"

"I don't know. You need to ask Dr. Karl."

"One more thing: do you have a plain pacemaker or a pacemaker-defibrillator?"

"I never heard of no defibrillator. I reckon it's just a regular pacemaker."

"That's good," I said.

I read the chart and examined him. His face and eyes were red and swollen, and there were chalky white opacities behind the pupils. He had a pacemaker under his left collarbone, the usual location, and his heart rate was rapid and irregular. The lining of his mouth was pale.

"You sure you don't have a defibrillator? You've never been given a shock or a jolt?" I asked.

"Nope. Never had that happen," Herschel said, firmly.

I scanned Karl's notes.

"So you're eighty, married, a rancher out in Hotspur County. You smoked a pack a day till seven years ago. You don't drink any alcohol. You were on metformin for diabetes but now you control it with diet alone. You take warfarin; I expect that's for atrial fibrillation. You've had prostate cancer, treated with chemo and radiation six years ago. You just had an upper endoscopy and colonoscopy by Dr. Wegener in Abilene ten days ago. Correct so far?"

"Yes, sir," Herschel nodded, and coughed.

"You sound congested."

"I'm allergic to cedar, and you know what's growing everywhere? Cedar!"

"When I examined you, your heart rate was rapid and irregular. It slows down and then speeds up. You have atrial fibrillation. Your heart rate is high. Are you taking a decongestant for your allergies?

"Yes."

"Decongestants can aggravate your atrial fibrillation."

"Don't know what that means, the heart deal, atrial whatever, but they tell me I got it."

"Atrial fibrillation means the upper, smaller chambers of your heart, called the atria, are not squeezing blood into the lower chambers. It's like they're shivering instead of squeezing. So the blood slows down in the atria. That's why it's called atrial fibrillation."

"What's wrong with that?"

"When blood slows down it's more likely to clot. If you do develop small clots, you could have a stroke."

"That's why I got to take warfarin? On account of the atrial whatever?"

"Exactly. Your risk of stroke goes up a lot, like thirty-five percent. But when you take a blood thinner like Coumadin, it reduces that extra risk down a lot."

"So I need to stay on the Warfarin forever?"

"Yes. It's protecting you from a stroke. But it's also aggravating your bleeding."

"I get it, Doc. Guess I'm screwed, huh? Cause if I stop Warfarin to stop the bleeding, I could end up with a big fat stroke!"

"That's correct, unfortunately."

"So what's the plan?"

"We just need to see what's going on and stop your bleeding. Then you can get back on Warfarin safely. I think you're bleeding from radiation damage and there's a special medicine I'm going to use to stop it."

Hershel shook his head.

"Doc Wegener couldn't fix it. They say he's the best."

"I read his notes. He hasn't tried this treatment."

"Doc Wegener told me he was top of his class in Yale or somewhere. Maybe he was fixing to start this new deal, too."

"I know he's a well-trained specialist, I'm sure he's brilliant," I mumbled without enthusiasm.

"What's this magic stuff you're going to give me?" Herschel asked.

"Formalin solution, four percent."

Herschel jerked back.

"What? Formalin? *Formalin?* That's what we used in the undertaking business. We inject it into dead bodies to stop them from rotting!"

"I know."

"But formalin is a poison!" Herschel cried.

Before I could answer, the door flew open and Hawkeye stormed in. His face was red and he was panting. He flung his bag into a corner, sat down heavily on a stool and turned to me.

"So what the hell is going on?" he bellowed.

"Don't blaspheme in here," Penny sang out from the corridor.

"Shut up! I want to know, what the hell, what the *heck*, is going on? When I signed up for this gig, I thought, okay, the pay's piss poor but at least there won't be emergencies. I mean, what can you guys do here? And yet you call me in for someone who's actively bleeding!"

"Karl called you in. He asked me to do the colonoscopy."

"Why are *you* doing the scope? It's Karl's patient," Hawkeye snapped.

Penny stepped in.

"Because *Dr. Mathur's* a specialist and *Dr. Karl* is a family physician. We've got Dr. Karl's patient, Mr. Herschel Dunn, here. Mr. Dunn has been bleeding so we need to scope him and fix it," she declared.

"What's his hemoglobin?" Hawkeye asked.

"Seven point two," Penny answered.

"Then give him a blood transfusion!"

"We just did," Penny replied, evenly.

"Send him to Abilene! What are you going to do here in this shitty little hospital? Ship him!"

"He's already been to Abilene. He saw the top GI specialist there and they diagnosed the problem but his treatment isn't working."

"What can we possibly do here that they couldn't?"

"Oh, don't underestimate us, Hockey. We can do unexpected things that will surprise you," Penny declared.

"That's what the bishop said to actress," he mumbled.

Penny was incensed.

"How dare you? I told you to never talk like that!" Penny boiled.

Hawkeye threw up his arms in surrender. Herschel turned towards Hawkeye.

"Actually, it's true. I've been to Abilene, sir. Saw Dr. Wegener."

"Dr. Wegener! He's the best. What did he say?" Hawkeye asked.

"He did an upper scope and a lower scope on me. Said I was bleeding from the radiation they done give me for my prostate cancer. He gave me some steroid to push up my butt and he burnt the radiation spots with a laser. But I'm still bleeding."

Hawkeye turned to me.

"Dr. Wegener! Wasn't he the one who screwed with you? Wouldn't even talk to you?"

"Yes."

Hawkeye rubbed his hands in glee.

"This is great! So now it's up to you, Wegener's archenemy, to find out what's happening. You really need to fix Herschel! Show Wegener that he missed the diagnosis or something. Find it and fix it so Wegener can just stick it up his ass!" Hawkeye chortled.

"Don't talk like that!" Penny protested.

"Oh, I'm so tired of all this! You and your fine manners and prissiness! I can barely open my mouth here!" Hawkeye complained.

I put my hand on Hawkeye's shoulder.

"Look, let's focus on Mr. Herschel and get started. Penny has a good IV going. Check his consents and do the time-out. Get your propofol, Hawkeye."

Hawkeye read the chart, asked a few questions, and slouched out. He returned with a medication box. He drew up two syringes of white fluid.

"Milk of amnesia, coming right up!" he drawled.

"No, stop!" Penny said. "I haven't done the time-out."

Hawkeye stiffened.

"Hurry up, nursey. Your IV doesn't look so good to me."

Penny glared at him. She spoke in a loud, clear voice.

"This is Herschel Dunn. His date of birth is July the 2nd, 1921, and he's eighty years old, allergic to sulfa, blood thinners have been held for five days, here for upper and lower endoscopy by Dr. Mathur."

"Dr. Becker just said colonoscopy. Did you want to do both upper and lower scopes?"

"Correct."

"Just to check for a hidden ulcer? In case Dr. Wegener missed something?"

"Yes," I said.

"I bet that would make your day!" Hawkeye said.

"Can we please stop talking and get started?" Penny asked, sharply.

Hawkeye snorted.

"Hold it. We can't get started. Your precious IV just blew, nursey. Give me a start kit, I'll have to get another," Hawkeye announced, with satisfaction. "Totally *useless* IV!"

"No! It was a good IV!" Penny protested.

"It's blown."

"No! Can't be!"

"Useless butterfly needle! Of course it's blown!"

"Shut the front door! It's not blown!" Penny insisted.

I looked at the IV. The tissue was swollen and the saline had stopped dripping.

"Sorry. It's blown," I said.

"Hah!" Hawkeye gloated and pulled out the butterfly needle and threw it into a sharps container. He swabbed Herschel's hand with alcohol and tied a tourniquet at the wrist.

Penny silently handed him an IV needle and starter kit. Hawkeye glanced at it and tossed it back to her.

"What the helicopter?" Penny cried out, angrily.

"I don't want another stupid butterfly needle, I want an 18 gauge Intracath! I don't want this one to blow as well! What's wrong with you?"

Penny started to say something but stopped. Hawkeye pounced.

"I'm sorry, were you going to say something or just open and close your mouth?" he inquired, acidly.

"You're extremely rude," Penny said.

Hawkeye ignored her. He rotated Herschel's hand and searched for a vein. He picked up the Intracath needle and shook off the plastic cover. He took a deep breath. Penny stepped closer.

"I know you're irritated about having to come in for this case but your attitude sucks," she hissed. Hawkeye ignored her.

"Big stick now!" he warned and slid the long needle smoothly into the vein. I saw a flashback of blood. Hawkeye whooped; Penny said nothing.

Hawkeye flushed the Intracath needle with saline.

"I'm in. Give me the IV," Hawkeye said, exhaling.

"Good job," Penny mumbled. She placed a hollow plastic bite block between Herschel's teeth.

"Mr. Herschel, this little piece of plastic protects your teeth from our scope and our scope from your teeth," she explained.

"I've given him a little lidocaine to numb the vein. Sometimes propofol can burn as it goes in. I'm giving him fifty milligrams." Hawkeye said.

Herschel closed his eyes. Hawkeye waited a few seconds and tickled

Herschel's eyelashes, then tapped him on the forehead. There was no response.

"All yours, Doc! Now, go find out what's broke and fix it."

I picked up the endoscope and tested it. I inserted the tip through the bite block into Herschel's mouth, then down his throat into his food pipe.

"I'm in the esophagus. I'm looking for swollen veins called varices. They can bleed and cause severe anemia," I said.

"Wouldn't the awesome Dr. Wegener have seen them?" Hawkeye asked.

"Yes," I admitted, "but if Herschel had lost a lot of blood they could have deflated and might not have been obvious."

I examined the esophagus closely.

"It looks normal. No swollen veins. Let me check the stomach now. I'm looking for ulcers and abnormal blood vessels."

I looked carefully. I washed the lining repeatedly and inflated the stomach with air. It was perfectly healthy.

"Looks good to me," Hawkeye said.

"Yes. It's normal," I agreed.

I advanced the tip of the instrument into the duodenum, the first part of the small intestine.

"See anything?" Hawkeye asked.

"Nothing abnormal. It looks fine."

"*Fine?* Are you sure?" Hawkeye persisted. "Look again, Doc."

I re-examined the duodenum and stomach.

"It all looks perfect. I can't find anything wrong. And he just had normal biopsies of the stomach, so we don't really need to repeat them."

Hawkeye was disappointed.

"Okay, Doc. I was hoping you'd find something but I guess Wegener didn't miss anything on the upper."

I nodded.

"Let's turn him around and check his rear end. He must be bleeding from there," I said.

We disconnected the leads and tubing and rotated the bed so that Herschel faced away from me. We reconnected everything and I picked up the colonoscope.

"Looks much bigger and meaner than the upper scope," Hawkeye noted.

"Yes, the colon is a large organ, at least five feet long, sometimes more than that."

"How can that be?" Penny objected. "The scope is less than five feet long."

"The scope telescopes the colon. The colon develops lots of folds as it gets pulled over the scope," I explained. "It's like putting your arm in a sleeve that's a little too long."

I examined the rectum with my finger. There was sticky red blood. I lubricated and inserted the tip of the colonoscope into the rectum. Bright red blood squirted out immediately. Herschel moaned and moved.

"Whoa, Doc! Man, that's a lot of blood just sitting there," Hawkeye said.

"Yes. It seems to be coming from something bleeding nearby," I said.

"How do you know that?" Penny questioned.

"The blood is liquid and bright red, so it hasn't had time to change color or harden into clots. That means the source of the bleeding is in or near the rectum."

I washed the front wall of the rectum right behind the prostate. There were a dozen bright red blood vessels, twisted, and covered with fine tendrils. They looked like a collection of red spiders. There were over twenty burn marks, small white scars like cigarette burns, on and in-between the corkscrew vessels.

"Those white scars are fresh scars from where Dr. Wegener cauterized them recently," I explained.

As we watched, an orange glaze developed and crimson drops formed over the blood vessels. The drops ballooned and dripped to form a small red puddle.

"No doubt about it, that sucker's bleeding!" Hawkeye boomed.

"I'm going to check the rest of the colon. There could be more than one source of bleeding," I said.

"Go for it, Doc! Try to find something good."

I didn't say anything.

"Doesn't it bother you, how Wegener always throws in that bit about being the top of his graduating class?" Hawkeye asked me.

"I'm just going to focus on the exam," I answered.

I advanced the scope gently through the left colon, across the transverse colon, slipped into the right colon, and quickly reached the end.

"Okay, I'm in the cecum. I also saw a couple of leaky blood vessels here and there, but nothing impressive."

"Is he bleeding from those?" Penny asked.

"No, they're not bleeding. I'm pulling back."

"So your enemy Dr. Wegener was right. He's bleeding from the radiation damage in the rectum," Hawkeye said.

"He's not my enemy."

"He's definitely not your friend! He wouldn't even talk to you!" Hawkeye pointed out.

"True. But I'm hopeful that I can talk to him and convince him that I'm no threat to him. In fact, I think that we could work together."

Hawkeye snorted.

"Yes, and we will all love everyone and we will all be happy and friendly together, forever and ever. La-la-la-lah!" he sang in falsetto. "Like that's *ever* going to happen."

"You are so nasty!" Penny said.

"I'm not nasty, I'm a *realist*. A realist, okay? Let me tell you something. Just because doctors have studied a lot doesn't make them nice people, okay? They can be real shits!" Hawkeye snapped.

"Doctors are just as good and bad as everyone else," I agreed.

"But everyone expects them to always be so good! I can tell you, they're just as mean as everyone else," Hawkeye said.

"Doctors are held to a different standard, that's true," I said.

"You got that right. But your deal with Dr. Wegener, I heard he wouldn't even talk to you and doesn't want you on staff at the hospital. Do you think he's racist?"

I shifted uncomfortably.

"Maybe I offended him," I said. "I prefer to think it's a professional issue, not racism."

Hawkeye appeared to have made up his mind. He shook his head from side to side, grinning.

"I've worked with doctors who are really shitty and mean. And racist," Hawkeye added, after a pause.

"I think Dr. Wegener is right about Herschel. Herschel is bleeding from radiation damage in the rectum. The medical term is radiation proctitis. But the bigger problem is figuring out how we can stop the bleeding."

"Can't you burn it with a laser?"

"Yes, that's an option. But Dr. Wegener just did it and it hasn't worked. Steroid enemas and suppositories have also been tried and they're not helping either."

"So what else can be done?" Hawkeye asked.

"There is another option. It's an unusual treatment, but it works. It's formalin, as a four percent solution, that we can spray into the rectum now and he can take enemas of the same formalin solution every night for two months. I've used it before on other patients and it really helps."

"The pharmacist just sent it up. You asked for three hundred cc of the four percent solution?" Penny said.

"Exactly. Just draw it up in a fifty cc syringe and I'll keep squirting it on the leaking blood vessels."

Penny looked uncomfortably at Hawkeye.

"Should we be doing this?" she wondered.

Hawkeye shrugged.

"I mean, formalin is a poison, right?" she said.

"Right. But we're using a very dilute amount to seal the leaky vessels and stop the bleeding," I explained.

Penny grasped my wrist.

"You *sure* it's safe?" she asked. "They use formalin in funeral homes to embalm dead bodies."

"I realize that. The same chemical has different uses at different strengths. We are using very weak formalin."

"Are you *really* sure?"

"I am. We used this a lot at the VA hospital in Houston where I trained. It works well. It's cheap and stops the bleeding." I said.

Penny still looked doubtful. She let go of my wrist.

"I don't want to lose my license," she said. "*Formalin?* It sounds dangerous."

"I've used it. It's safe."

"How come Dr. Wegener didn't use it?"

I held up my hand.

"Okay, enough. This is a standard treatment. It just *sounds* weird. Remember, we make hydrochloric acid in our stomachs, and that's stronger than what we're using now."

"But, *Formalin?*" Penny shook her head.

"I take full responsibility." I said.

Penny looked at Hawkeye. He looked back dispassionately.

"He's the specialist," he shrugged.

Penny sighed and drew up the formalin solution. I squirted it gently into the rectum. After filling up the rectum, I rolled up a towel and held it against the anus.

"You're doing that so he doesn't blow it all out?" Penny asked.

"Yes."

"How long are you going to wait?" Hawkeye asked, wearily.

"Five or ten minutes."

"Oh, sweet Jesus!" Hawkeye groaned. "This is taking too long!"

Penny wagged her finger at him.

"Don't take the Lord's name in vain!" she hissed.

Hawkeye glared at me.

"Women!" he snarled. "Can't live *with* them, can't live *with* them!"

"You mean, can't live *with* them, can't live *without* them," Penny sniffed.

"Actually, no. I said exactly what I wanted to say," Hawkeye said, curtly.

"You said it wrong, Hockey. You said, can't live with them, can't live *with* them. You got it wrong. You should have said, women: can't live with them, can't live *without* them," Penny corrected.

"No, it was deliberate. I meant that women like you are seriously irritating. So believe me when I say, women, can't live with them, can't live *with* them!"

"You're a rude little man," Penny said, lowering her voice. "No wonder you're getting a divorce."

We waited in silence for five minutes. I kept the formalin solution in the rectum by maintaining firm pressure on the anus. I tried to break the ice.

"Anyone have plans for the weekend?" I asked.

"No," Penny snapped.

Hawkeye said nothing.

"Anyone tried Torchy's Tacos in Abilene? I've heard it's really good," I continued.

No response.

"Do you have a Torchy's in San Angelo, Hawkeye?"

Still no response. I waited a minute

"What's your favorite restaurant in San Angelo, Hawkeye?"

"Thai. Or Vietnamese."

"There may be one of those in Abilene," I said, a little too cheerfully.

Hawkeye turned to Penny.

"So, Miss Precious Penny, have you heard of the new Vietnamese restaurant in San Angelo?" he said, silkily.

"No," Penny said, warily.

"You know that they make a soup called Pho. It's written p-h-o but pronounced Fah," Hawkeye continued.

I knew where Hawkeye was headed. I closed my eyes and braced myself.

"So this new Vietnamese restaurant opens up and guess what they call it? They call it the Pho King!" Hawkeye smirked. "Seriously!"

"Hockey! Stop it!" Penny shrieked.

"They have a daily surprise dish. They call it, *what the Pho?*"

Penny turned to me.

"He can't talk like that! Make him stop talking like that!" she pleaded.

Hawkeye had one last line before I interjected.

"They have take-away. That's called *Pho-off!*"

I tried not to smile.

"You can't talk like that, Hawkeye! It's offensive," I declared. Hawkeye scowled.

A few minutes later, I removed the towel. Red-tinged water trickled out.

"Hey! There's a lot less bleeding!" Hawkeye noted.

"That's a good start. He will need to do these enemas three times a day."

"Great. Are we finally done?" Hawkeye asked, brusquely.

"Yes."

"Thank you, Jesus!"

Penny glared at him again.

"Doc, his wife is waiting outside. She went back home to get the reports from Dr. Wegener and to get Herschel's catheter," she said.

"He didn't tell me he had difficulty passing urine," I said.

I wiped the scope and suctioned cleaning enzymes through the channels and handed the instrument to Penny. I thanked her and Hawkeye, removed my gown and gloves, washed my hands, and stepped outside.

Florence Dunn was a short, wizened lady. She, too, had short white hair and large glasses hanging on a necklace. She wore a turtleneck pullover and jeans. We shook hands and introduced ourselves.

"Herschel told me you came to the house when he was sick with pneumonia last year. I was away in Alabama, visiting my folks. Thank you for coming out to see him," she said. "I didn't think doctors made home visits any more."

"I'm glad to help. He was pretty sick but we got him over that."

Florence nodded.

"I know Bill Hennessy went and got you, bless his heart, and you came on down and fixed him. Now we need you to help fix this darn bleeding," she continued. "What's causing the bleeding?"

"Mrs. Dunn, the radiation he received for prostate cancer damaged the lining of the rectum and the lining is bleeding. The bleeding is made worse by his warfarin, which is a blood thinner."

"Can we stop the blood thinner, Doctor?"

"He needs to stay on the blood thinner or else he could have a stroke."

"My lands! We don't want a stroke! His mother died of a stroke!"

"I saw the burn marks of the laser that Dr. Wegener had used and I know that he gave you steroid enemas as well."

"Durn right! Those steroid enemas, they're really high-dollar! Luckily the VA picked up most of the tab. They kind of helped in the beginning, but the bleeding came right back."

I paused.

"There is one treatment that's a little unusual. It's a standard treatment, but not one that we use all the time."

"What is it? We'll try anything!"

"Four percent formalin solution," I said, quietly.

She was taken aback.

"We use formalin in the embalming business! It's a nasty poison!" she cried.

"I agree, it's an unusual treatment. But it is well recognized and it does work. In fact, I just used it on Herschel and it stopped the bleeding."

She looked at me.

"Are you sure about this?"

I nodded slowly.

"You're not going to hurt my Herschel?"

I shook my head. Florence regarded me for a few minutes.

"I know you made a mistake on one of them colonoscopies," she said.

I turned red.

"Yes, that's true. There was a perforation. I've done thousands of colonoscopies and that was my first one ever."

Florence stared at me for a minute, then smiled.

"Had to happen here in a small town where everyone knows about it, huh?" she chuckled.

"No secrets in a small town," I shrugged.

"All right. Let's try the formalin."

"Where should I call it in?" I asked.

"Herschel uses both Owl Drugs and Tyson Drugs," Penny said.

"Jim at Owl Drugs had promised to compound it. So let's go with him."

"Okay. See now, I'm going to trust you on this formalin deal," Florence said, warily.

The OR door burst open and Hawkeye charged out, swinging his bag. He stopped to slap me on the shoulder.

"Hey, I just thought of another great benefit of the formalin. If he doesn't make it, you've already prepared his body for the funeral!" he boomed, and scuttled off.

Florence gazed after him

"I don't like that man," she muttered.

I took Florence back to the recovery room.

"I have a couple of concerns, Miss Florence. Herschel has bad cataracts and needs to get them removed," I said.

"How do you know?" Florence asked.

"When I went into the operating room, he couldn't recognize my face, even though the room was bright. His eye lenses are a thick white color and that means cataracts."

"Okay, thank you."

"I also think he is taking allergy medicines with decongestants for his allergies."

"He has bad allergies to cedar. He does take some pills for it."

"In older men, anti-allergy meds can make it difficult to pee and can cause a rapid heart beat."

Florence looked back at me with a smile.

"How did you know he's having a hard time peeing? I can't believe he told you."

"You went home to get his catheter. That means he's having a hard time peeing."

"So what should I do?"

"Tell him to stop using the anti-allergy meds. The urinary problems will get a lot better."

"Herschel believes in you. Ever since you and Bill Hennessy got him face down on the coffee table and whacked on his chest and got that corruption out, he believes in you!"

"Yes, I did a little bit of thumping to shake the infection out of his chest," I recalled.

"Worked like a charm. The reason Herschel didn't come back to you, we were tight for money. Just got through paying bills for the prostate cancer treatments."

"Didn't the VA pay?"

"Yes, but we had to get him to Albuquerque and that was expensive! Then the bleeding made him depressed. He just drips blood in his shorts and even his pants and everywhere."

"Have you tried diapers?"

Florence shook her head.

"He's too proud. Too proud to wear diapers."

"I understand. Hopefully, the bleeding will get a lot less. Also Herschel is low in blood, he's anemic. He needs to increase his iron tablets to twice daily, with meals and orange juice."

"Why? He's been on an iron pill for over a month!"

"You only absorb six percent of the iron you take in. You waste ninety-four percent. So you have to take it for a long time."

"I didn't know that. Why orange juice?"

"It improves absorption of the iron. So increase the iron to twice daily, with orange juice, and stay on it for another three months at least."

I handed her a report.

"This is a written summary of what I found and what I want Herschel to do. It's in plain language, no medical jargon. I'm going to make a copy of Dr. Wegener's report for my files."

"Thank you. I'm glad you've written it down. It's hard to remember everything."

I called the prescription to Owl Drugs. The pharmacist, Elvis Caldwell, was surprised.

"Don't get to compound this stuff often. A four percent solution of formalin, right?"

"Correct. Please instruct him to squirt it up into his rectum and then try to retain it there, not let it run out."

Elvis coughed.

"He's a mighty private man. He's going to hate shoving stuff up his hiney. But if that's what it takes to stop the bleeding, he'll do it, by golly. Still, he might refuse."

"He refused to come to the hospital when he was down with pneumonia last year."

"I know. Big Bill Hennessy grabbed you and got you to go do a home visit," Elvis chuckled. "Herschel refused to go with his wife to Alabama, because he refuses to fly. You know why he refuses to fly?"

"No."

"He has this prostate problem. So once, when he went to pee in the plane toilet, what with all the turbulence and all, he kind of missed the target. Well, the air hostess came after him and chewed him out! He was so embarrassed! So now he refuses to fly."

"How do you know all this?" I asked.

"No secrets in a small town," Elvis declared. "Reckoned you'd have figured that out by now."

CHAPTER 16

THE WOMAN WHO KEPT ON BLEEDING

"Hello, hello, hello, Doctor!" Simon voice boomed over the phone.

"Simon! Why are you calling me? I'm not on call, Karl - Dr. Becker - is on call."

"I know that, Doctor," Simon said.

"I'm working with my daughter Anjali on a school project. I have to finish it tonight."

"I realize this is terrible timing. I'm so *very* sorry to bother you, sir. But we've got one of your patients in here, a young lady by the name of Patricia White. She's come in with severe bleeding. Dr. Becker asked if you might see her as she might need an urgent endoscopy to check her for bleeding."

I was flustered.

"But I have to finish this project! It's due in school tomorrow morning. It can't wait."

"The way this young lady looks, she may not make it till the morning either," Simon said.

I groaned.

"Where is she bleeding from?" I asked.

"She's been throwing up blood and stomach contents for over eight hours now. Threw up a whole bunch of bright red blood about fifteen minutes ago in the parking lot. All her clothes are reeking of bile and vomit and blood."

"Can we transfer her to Abilene?"

"No beds available."

"How about San Angelo?"

"Same thing."

"Did you try both hospitals in Abilene?"

"Yes. And both hospitals in San Angelo."

"Can we send her to Dallas?"

"She's too unstable to transport her that far. Dr. Becker says no."

My mind raced over the possibilities.

"She has a history of alcohol and drug abuse. We need to check some labs to see if she has cirrhosis of the liver," I said.

"Can you tell that on a blood test?" Simon asked.

"Yes, but indirectly. We check the platelet count. If it's pretty low then we can predict that there's some degree of cirrhosis," I answered. "And we need the hemoglobin. Also, get a chemistry panel. We need to check the urea level."

"You got it. Want me to call Penny and Hawkeye? In case you're going to scope her for the bleeding?"

"No. If she's bleeding badly then we need to send her to the ICU in Abilene. When patients bleed from varices, they can lose a lot of blood very quickly. She needs to be in an ICU. Definitely not here."

"They don't have any beds. I just asked."

"Let's stabilize her and check again. Maybe a bed will open up."

"I will call the hospitals again, Doctor. Will you please come to see her?"

I paused. I looked at my watch.

"Yes. I'll be there soon. Five minutes. I'll come in quickly, assess her and ship her to Abilene. Then I can get back and finish Anjali's art project. Get that blood count and full chemistry panel stat."

Patricia White was gaunt. She was jaundiced and hunched unsteadily over a plastic basin. She retched and spat a string of blood into it. She didn't look up.

"Patty! I haven't seen you in ages!" I said.

"Been busy," she mumbled.

"You look really weak."

"I feel terrible. I've been sick to my stomach. Started throwing up blood this morning."

"Was the throw-up bright red or dark brown?"

"At first it was bright red, then brown."

"Any pain?"

"Nah. Just some cramping."

"Any black colored stools?"

"Yeah. Two really black stools. Black, like tar. Liquid stools, they were."

"Are you feeling dizzy?"

"Yeah. I can't really stand up. Feels like I'm going to pass out."

Simon handed me her chart and I scanned it. I examined her quickly.

"Patty, your blood pressure is eighty by sixty, and your pulse is ninety-eight per minute. You're jaundiced, which means your skin is yellow because your liver is damaged."

"What? My liver is damaged?"

"Yes. It's probably from alcohol. Have you been drinking?"

Patty shrugged. She had red spots over her upper chest and on both sides of her nose. Her hands trembled, but there was no smell of alcohol.

"I think you've been drinking." I said.

"You always say that."

"Patty, your skin is yellow. You've developed these little red spots over your face and upper chest and they weren't there the last time I saw you. They're called spider nevi, or just spiders."

I read her chart quickly.

"So how much are you drinking?" I asked.

"Same as usual. Maybe a bit more since Jerry left town."

"You're drinking more than usual."

"How can you tell?"

"Besides the fresh crop of red spiders on your chest, your whole face has a red flush. Your salivary glands are enlarged. Your hands are trembling."

"But she doesn't smell of alcohol." Simon pointed out.

Patty turned to me, triumphantly.

"True. But she might be drinking vodka. Vodka doesn't make your breath smell. Preferred by all the serious alcoholics."

Patty was deflated.

"Now I'm going to examine you," I said.

I inspected her fingers and her hands, listened to her heart and lungs and palpated her abdomen. I quickly checked her knee and ankle reflexes and tested for sensation in her face, arms and legs.

I straightened up and addressed Patty.

"Besides the jaundice, your liver is enlarged and tender, and your spleen is swollen as well," I said. "Simon, get me the lab results. I'm going to transfer her to Abilene."

"I already called. Dr. Wegener is on call at both hospitals and he's busy with an emergency case. He said he doesn't know when he can call back."

"Did you tell him that it was my patient?"

"Yes. Sorry."

I groaned.

"We have a history. We don't get along. How about San Angelo?"

"They won't take her. They said the last time they accepted her she ended up suing them."

I turned to Patty in surprise.

"Yes. I did! They were really mean to me! They let an IV infiltrate into my forearm and it swelled up like a balloon. It crushed the nerves and blood vessels and cut off the blood into my hand and they were saying, we may need to cut your arm off! So, yeah, I sued the crap out of them."

"So where else can we send her?" I asked aloud.

"We can try Dallas Presbyterian or Harris Methodist," Simon suggested.

Suddenly there was a stench of rotting blood and feces. Patty moaned and slumped. A pool of reddish-black liquid formed rapidly under her.

"Turn her to her side!" I ordered. "See how much blood she's losing!"

"She's just pouring out her rear end!" Simon said.

"Do you have a good IV in her?"

"Yes, I've got an eighteen gauge in her left hand."

"Get another on the right side. Give her normal saline wide open. We've got to get her blood pressure up!"

I laid Patricia on her side and lowered the head end of the bed. I strapped on a blood pressure cuff and applied chest leads to monitor her heart rhythm. Simon clipped a pulse oximeter on her earlobe.

"Her blood pressure is dropping!" Simon said.

"Give her fluids and keep her head low. What was her hemoglobin on admission?" I asked.

"Eight point four. But she's thrown up since then, so it's probably lower now."

Patty groaned loudly and a fresh wave of magenta liquid shot out and flooded the gurney behind her hips. Simon rushed to cover it up with towels but it was too late. The thick red tar poured onto the floor, splattering him.

"Good Lord!" Simon cried and tried to avoid the spray of blood and feces.

"Just cover it up with towels. We need that second IV now and get me two units of O negative blood stat!"

Simon threw towels on the gurney and on the floor beneath. He rushed off to the nurses' station to get the blood. I started another IV line. Patricia stirred and reached for my wrist.

"I don't think I'm going to make it this time," she mumbled.

"Nonsense! You're going to be fine."

"No, I can tell this is different. I feel like I'm not really here, like I'm floating."

"That's because you've lost so much blood that your brain has become confused. Patty, I don't see a vein on your right side."

"I figured you were going to say that. I used 'em all up when I was doing drugs."

"I need to start a central line in your neck."

"Like you did a couple years ago?"

"Right. Do you remember when you had that infection in your blood stream? It had infected your heart and even one of your eyes. It was called a Roth spot."

"Yeah, I remember. I had doctors and medical students coming to check out my eye all the time."

I slipped on a mask, gloves, and a gown. I cleaned Patty's neck with iodine and wiped it with alcohol. I draped sterile green towels all around the right side of her neck, leaving only a small area the size of a pack of cards exposed. I put on a pair of sterile gloves over the regular ones and opened a central line kit.

"Okay, I'm pulling up a stool so I can sit down and then I'm going to inject some lidocaine into your neck."

"Go for it, Doc," she croaked.

I palpated the carotid artery in the neck with the fingertips of my left hand and used a small five cc syringe and needle to locate the internal jugular vein. I then changed to a larger needle and used the same angle and location to access the jugular vein. I advanced a guide wire through the large needle and down into the vein.

"Did you get it?" Patty whispered.

"Yes."

"Hallelujah!" Patty said.

"Do you remember what you told me when I got into your neck vein two years ago?"

"Nope."

"You said, *hey, you must be good, Doc, because I've been trying to hit that one for weeks!*"

"So what?"

"The thought of you standing in front of a mirror and jabbing yourself with a big dirty needle, that was too much."

"Well, at least I ain't doing IV no more," Patty said, softly.

Simon returned, holding on to two bags of blood. He kept one in a small water heater and connected the other to Patty's IV.

"Sorry for the delay. Had to find the heater. How fast should I give the blood?"

"Run it in wide open," I ordered.

Simon hesitated.

"Won't that overload her?" he asked.

"Not at all. She's really dehydrated and has lost so much blood already."

"If you're sure," Simon hesitated.

"Right now we've got to get her blood pressure up! Give the blood wide open!"

Simon turned up the drip and blood streamed out.

"I called Abilene again, Dr. Mathur, and Dr. Wegener is still tied up. He told the nursing supervisor he was too busy talk to you."

I nodded.

"I'm going to stitch this central line into her neck and I'm going to call the nursing supervisor myself. This is crazy! I've applied for consulting privileges at Abilene Memorial. If they had approved me, I could have admitted Patty myself!"

"Her cell number is by the phone in the dictation room."

I quickly stitched the new IV line into the skin of the neck. Patty didn't flinch. I thought back two years ago when she had bacterial endocarditis, a dangerous infection of the bloodstream, caused by using dirty needles to inject drugs.

"You're faster than you were last time," Patty said.

"Thanks. Do you need to poop again?"

"No."

"Good. Then maybe the bleeding has slowed down. I'm going to talk to the nursing supervisor and see if I can transfer you to the ICU there."

"Can you do that?"

"I applied for admitting privileges over a month ago. I haven't heard anything. Maybe they approved it and just haven't told me."

I removed the towels and plastic around her neck and connected saline to the neck IV.

"Simon! Get Ted to shoot a plain x-ray of the neck and upper chest stat! I need to make sure it's safe to use it."

"Will do, Doctor."

I called from the dictation room.

"Hello! Abilene Hospital. This is Sue Smart, nursing supervisor."

"Hello. This is Dr. Mathur in Hotspur. I'm an internist and gastroenterologist. I have a young lady with suspected variceal bleeding. She has cirrhosis of the liver. I've started blood for her but she needs an ICU bed."

"Who is the accepting physician?"

"Well, Dr. Wegener is in an emergency and can't answer me. I've applied for privileges and may have been approved. I wanted to admit her under myself."

"Have you received an appointment letter, Doctor?"

"No. I applied for privileges a month ago. Maybe they granted them already. Can you check?"

"Sure. Let me place you on a brief hold while I call administration."

I stepped back into the emergency room.

"Any more bleeding?"

"No. So far so good," Simon said.

I returned to the phone. Within minutes Sue was back.

"Doctor, I called the administrator on call. Your application has been reviewed but not approved yet. In fact, the medical executive committee is meeting tomorrow at noon and your application is on the agenda."

"But what about right now?"

"I'm sorry. You will have to involve someone who already has admitting privileges here."

I sighed. I thanked Sue and hung up. I turned to Simon.

"So I have to ask Dr. Wegener, but he's busy. So should I talk to someone in the Abilene ER to accept my patient?"

Simon shook his head.

"That won't help because they would still need Dr. Wegener to accept the patient. They can't help without Dr. Wegener's approval," he said.

"So should I look at Abilene Baptist Hospital instead?"

"Won't help. Dr. Wegener is on call for gastroenterology at both hospitals," Simon said.

"Try Dallas again," I ordered. "I'm going to call the hospitals in Lubbock."

* * *

I had no success. I gave up and stepped back into the emergency room. To my surprise, Penny was setting up the mobile cart, screen and upper endoscope. I turned to Simon.

"I figured you would want to scope her and stop the bleeding, so I called Penny and Hawkeye. I thought that's what you would want. Penny's here but I haven't seen Hawkeye," Simon said.

"Thank you. You're exactly right. I need to scope her and stop any further bleeding before she starts up again. I guess I should tell my daughter I won't be home till later."

"Sorry," Patty mumbled.

"Where's Hawkeye?"

"He's not answering his phone. But there's a bad patch between San Angelo and Hotspur where you can't get a signal."

"I'm worried that Patty has blood in her stomach. So when we sedate her to look down her throat and do the endoscopy, she might upchuck a lot of blood. It could get sucked into her lungs."

"So should we hold off the endoscopy?" Penny asked.

"No. We don't have any more blood. It will take at least three hours to get her to Dallas or Fort Worth. She could bleed out. We've got to do something *right now*."

"I feel sick, like I need to throw up," Patty said, raising herself on an elbow. She retched and brought up a small blood clot.

Simon wiped her face and hands with a wet towel and changed her sheets. He cleaned the tarry blood off Patty's buttocks and legs. He gently separated her thighs and scrubbed off the matted blood.

"Thank you, darling, I'll do that for you some day," Patty croaked. Simon flushed.

"Patty, I need to explain something to you. You've got a lot of blood in your stomach and I need to stop the bleeding. You could bleed to death. We have to look inside your stomach," I explained.

Patty was alarmed.

"When do you want to do this?" she asked.

"I need to get started right now. We will have to intubate you to protect your lungs," I said.

"What do you mean?" she said.

"Patty, your stomach has a lot of blood. When I sedate you, you might throw up some of that blood. It could get sucked into your lungs and cause pneumonia."

"So what are you going to do?"

"I'm going to put a small plastic tube into your lungs. We will push oxygen in and out of your lungs for you. The tube will protect your airway and will prevent blood from getting into your airways and lungs."

Patty shuddered.

"It sounds scary. Will you put me to sleep first?" she asked. "I don't want to feel anything."

"Of course. But I don't want to sedate you too much or paralyze you before I place that tube in your lungs."

"Why not? I just told you, I don't want to feel anything!"

I paused.

"Patty, if I knock you out and then I can't get a tube into your lungs, we're in big trouble. Then I've stopped your breathing and I can't help you get oxygen."

"Have you done this before?"

"Yes. Many times."

"Have you ever failed to get the tube in?"

"No."

"Then I'll take my chances. Do your best."

"I will. Simon, get me a seven endotracheal tube and a Mackintosh blade. Get me ten of midazolam."

"Do you want a muscle paralyzing agent?" Simon asked.

"No, too dangerous. If I paralyze her, she could stop breathing and there's no antidote. But with midazolam, there is an antidote. We can use romazicon. Draw up two milligrams of romazicon."

Simon hesitated.

"We have a problem. The romazicon is past the expiry date."

I groaned.

"How far out are we?"

"Two months."

"Draw it up anyway. Two months isn't too bad. I've read where these medicines can be good for two years after the expiry date. Let's hope we won't need the antidote."

I made Patty lie flat and inserted a pillow under her shoulders. Her head fell back and she looked straight at me, quivering. I suctioned her mouth dry. I changed gowns, gloves and face shield and stood above her head. She looked shaky.

"I'm really scared, Doc," she whispered.

"Don't worry, it's going to be just fine," I said.

"Ready with the midazolam," Simon announced.

"Give her two and a half milligrams now."

Simon injected the medicine. We waited two minutes.

"I don't feel anything," Patty said.

"Another two point five," I ordered.

We watched the pulse oximeter and the heart monitor.

"Her oxygen is down to ninety percent but she looks pretty awake," Simon said.

"I'm awake, Doc, I'm awake! Give me some more juice," Patty mumbled.

"Give her another two milligrams," I said.

Patty finally relaxed. Her eyes closed, her jaws went loose and her shoulders slumped. I grabbed the Mackintosh blade with my right hand and opened her mouth with my left. Patty immediately woke up and struggled. I put the Mackintosh down.

"Okay. She's not ready. Another two of midazolam."

Simon hesitated.

"Her oxygen's down to eighty-eight percent. You sure, Doctor?"

"We've got to go ahead. The alcohol abuse makes her liver just chew up the midazolam."

"Her oxygen's now down to eighty five percent!"

"I realize that."

I grasped her jaw and pulled her mouth open. She moved a little. I slid the blade of the Mackintosh forceps over her tongue and stopped just above the vocal cords. I saw the larynx and motioned to Simon. He handed me the endotracheal tube.

Before I could slide the tube in, Patty coughed loudly. A spray of blood and phlegm splattered my face shield. I retreated and wiped it clean.

"At least I saw the vocal cords. I'm going to get it in. I just have to sedate her a little more."

"Not only is her oxygen down to eighty three percent, Doctor, her blood pressure's dropping! It's now ninety by fifty."

"Could be because of all the midazolam I've given her. Give her one more milligram."

Simon hesitated, then pushed the last milligram.

I waited thirty seconds, then opened Patty's mouth and suctioned it clear. I replaced the Mackintosh and pulled up hard. The vocal cords popped into view. I held my breath and motioned for the tube.

Simon dropped it on the floor.

"Oh crap!" he swore. He rushed to the dictation room to find another one. I withdrew the Mackintosh and cursed.

"I am so *very* sorry!" he cried, as he returned with another tube.

"That's okay," I said through gritted teeth

Two alarms went off.

"Her blood pressure's down to eighty systolic and her heart rate's dropping! You should stop!" Simon said.

"Just give me the tube. Press down on her neck a little, and stop telling me what the monitor says!" I snapped.

I opened her mouth again. There was no resistance this time. I slid in the Mackintosh and lifted up forcefully. Frothy phlegm had collected in her throat and obscured the vocal cords.

"Do you want suction, doctor?"

A third alarm went off.

"No! She's stopped breathing and her heart's shutting down! There's no time! I'm going in blind."

I thrust the tube deeply. I saw it hit the side of the larynx. I pulled back and angulated the tip and tried again. It slid right in, past the vocal cords. I whooped and quickly inflated the balloon that held it in place.

"I'm pretty sure I'm in!" I said. I quickly connected the tube to an oxygen bag and Simon squeezed it. Patty's chest rose and fell. I listened to both sides of her chest.

"I can hear good air entry bilaterally. I'm in, I'm sure of it. Let's get ready for the endoscopy. Simon, you need to keep bagging her. About two squeezes every ten seconds but watch the monitor."

"Do you want a chest X-ray to confirm position of the tube?"

"No, there's no time."

"But Dr. Becker always does that."

"Thank you. No!"

"It's for the patient's safety," Simon protested.

"I know. But right now, we don't have time. It will take Ted thirty minutes to come and shoot an X-ray and get us the film. I don't have the time. I can hear breath sounds on both sides. I'm going with that."

Simon nodded.

"Her oxygen has come up nicely, it's already ninety-two percent," he conceded. "Maybe we won't need the X-ray."

Penny handed me the scope. She had set up the screen so that it was right in front of me.

"Do you want me to turn her onto her left side?" she asked.

"No, leave her on her back. I'm starting now."

I placed the tip of the endoscope in the mouth and guided it past the endotracheal tube, and into the food pipe. The screen immediately turned bright red.

"The food pipe is full of blood. See these large swollen veins with red marks? She's bleeding from these swollen veins. They're called varices."

"Kind of like varicose veins, but in the food pipe?" Simon wondered.

"Exactly. The liver cirrhosis causes blood to back up in the veins of the food pipe or esophagus, and they swell up and burst and bleed. So we've made the diagnosis. She's got bleeding esophageal varices."

"That's a lot of blood!" Penny said.

I advanced the scope.

"Yes. Now I'm checking the stomach, which is also full of blood."

"Good thing you intubated her," Penny said.

"No ulcers in the stomach or intestine. Just a lot of old blood. I'm checking the roof of the stomach for swollen veins."

"You're looking for varices in the stomach?"

"Yes."

"Could they bleed as well?"

"Yes. Luckily, she doesn't have them. Those can bleed really badly and are very hard to control."

"Are you going to do some treatment for the bleeding?" Penny asked.

"Absolutely! I'm going to pull out and put a banding apparatus on the scope. Then I'm going to put some rubber bands on the bleeding veins and pinch them closed."

I withdrew the scope completely. Penny and I assembled a band applicator on the scope. Simon watched keenly. We connected a plastic barrel to the tip of the scope and pulled a trip wire through the scope. It emerged near the controls.

"So that apparatus at the tip is a little barrel with rubber bands that have been stretched," Simon observed. "And you release the bands by pulling on the wire?"

"Correct."

"But how do you get the rubber bands onto the veins?"

"You go to the base of the vein and suck the tissue into the barrel. Then you pull the trip wire to release the bands one at a time," I explained.

The door opened and Hawkeye stumbled in. He froze.

"*What!* You started without me?" he wailed. "I came all this way!"

"Where were you? Dr. Mathur had to intubate the patient!" Penny said.

"We were waiting on you," Simon said. "We were all waiting on you."

"As it should be," Hawkeye sneered. "Give me that."

He moved to the patient's head and took over the oxygen bag.

"So what kept you, Hockey?" Penny persisted.

"If you must know, I hit a deer. I was doing eighty, maybe eighty-five miles and this big doe just ran onto the road. She saw me coming, she was way off the road and then suddenly decided to rush across! I couldn't avoid her. She blew out my headlamp and smashed up the front of my Beemer! God, I'm so pissed!"

"Don't blaspheme!" Penny warned.

"Oh, shut up!"

Hawkeye pulled a stethoscope out of his bag and listened for air movement in both lungs. He nodded and continued bagging her.

"Go ahead. You're in good position. How much have you given her?" he asked.

"Ten of midazolam."

"Ten! Wow, that's a lot. Any paralytics?"

"No."

"Any narcotics?"

"No. I wanted to be safe. Just in case I wasn't able to get the tube in."

Hawkeye nodded.

"I'm going to do the band ligation now," I warned

"In that case, hold on. Let me give her a little morphine. That band ligation can hurt and I don't want her waking up," Hawkeye said.

Simon jumped to the door.

"We don't have any morphine here. I'll have to go get it. Back in a jiffy," Simon said. He rushed off to the pharmacy. The three of us waited.

"You know what you need, Hockey?" Penny said, brightly.

"I don't need your advice," Hawkeye growled.

"You need a pet. You're too tense."

"When I want your opinion, I'll give it to you, okay?"

"I have a cat, Pandora, she's the queen of the house. She snuggles up to me and squeezes in next to me when I sleep."

"Oh, spare me," Hawkeye moaned.

"She isn't fussy. She just loves on me. She takes care of herself, bless her heart."

Hawkeye was irritated.

"Penny, has having a cat helped you, made you calm?" I intervened.

"Yes, always. Well, not always. Sometimes I get aggravated. Like the other day, I worked on a jigsaw puzzle all night and the next morning Pandora had messed it all up! I was so upset with her!"

Hawkeye snorted.

"The jigsaw puzzle was on the table?" he asked.

"No, I did it on the floor. And when I woke up, it was all broken up and there was cat hair everywhere!" Penny complained.

Hawkeye was scathing.

"What did you expect? You leave a jigsaw puzzle half done on the floor where your cat can mess it up and then you're surprised the next day when she did just that?" he snapped.

"I didn't expect it," Penny countered.

"What *did* you expect? Did you expect that you would wake up and the jigsaw puzzle would be completed and Pandora would be standing up, leaning against the wall, smoking a cigar, and saying *you're welcome, bitch?*"

"Hawkeye! You can't talk like that!" I protested.

Penny was speechless. Her mouth fell open. Before she could respond, Simon rushed in.

"Here's the morphine. I drew up four milligrams," Simon said, waving a syringe. "Sorry it took so long. I had to sign out for it. Did I miss anything?"

Hawkeye chuckled and injected the morphine. Penny's face was red and swollen. I resumed the procedure rapidly.

"I'm inserting the scope again. Now I'm at the base of the biggest vein and I'm going to suction it up into the barrel and release a band on it," I explained.

I repeated the banding four times. Each time there was a spurt of blood and Penny recoiled. I pulled the scope back and waited.

"Look, the bleeding is slowing down," I pointed out.

We watched in silence. "Now I'm examining the stomach. There's a lot of old blood here, but no fresh blood. No other source of bleeding."

"That's a relief."

"I've checked the duodenum and there's old blood there, nothing fresh and no active bleeding there. I'm pulling out."

I withdrew the scope slowly. The bands on the varices were holding and the bleeding had stopped. I removed the scope completely and wiped it down. Penny took down the monitor, unplugged the cart, and wheeled the equipment out. She didn't say a word.

"Not like Penny to remain so quiet," Simon noted.

Hawkeye grasped the endotracheal tube.

"You're done, right?" he asked.

I nodded. He deflated the balloon of the endotracheal tube and gently eased it out of Patty's airway. He raised the head end of the bed and wiped her face. He suctioned her mouth again. Soon she was fully awake.

"Patty, we're all done. I'm going to admit you to the hospital and watch you. I will try Dallas Presbyterian and see if they can take you. At least you're stable now. You've had two units of blood and I've stopped the bleeding for now. I'm going to start a drip of octreotide and give you some antibiotics and get you to an ICU as fast as I can."

Patty nodded groggily.

I was starting to feel drowsy too. I went to the dictation room and finished my notes. I called Dallas Presbyterian and left messages for the on-call gastroenterologist. As I left, Patty grasped my hand.

"Sorry I messed up your daughter's art project."

I had forgotten about it. Guilt overwhelmed me.

"That's okay," I mumbled.

"It's not okay. She goes to St. John's, right?"

I nodded.

"Yes. They're pretty strict. Maybe they'll give her an extra day or two to complete the project," I said.

"Thank you, Doc. Thanks for helping me again."

"You're welcome."

Patty hesitated.

"I got no insurance, Doc."

"I know."

"I can't pay."

"I know."

"I hate that you had to leave your family to help me."

I was silent.

"You're a great doctor!"

I nodded.

Her words seemed so hollow, the victory so shallow. I realized that helping Patty was the right thing to do, but I should have anticipated emergencies and completed Anjali's project well before the deadline. I enjoyed spending time with my family and I was equally fond of medicine. I realized I spent more time and effort being a doctor than a father, and it saddened me. I recalled Priya innocently telling me that she always remembers me as being *a doctor*. I burned with shame. I have reduced clinic hours, reduced my call, and scheduled more time off, but to this day, I struggle to find that balance.

CHAPTER 17
THE MEDICAL EXECUTIVE COMMITTEE

Karl pounced as I walked into the office the next morning.

"Your Highness! Thank you for seeing Patty White last night."

"You're welcome."

Karl was grinning from ear to ear.

"I've got some big news for you. Get you a donut and some coffee. Let's go to that little conference room we got."

He handed me my steel coffee cup that said *Shit Specialist*. I filled it with coffee and broke a donut in half. Karl laughed and picked up two and waved me out of the office.

"Oh, come on! You can eat a whole donut," he protested.

"No, I can't. I have the five-six curse," I said.

"What's that?"

"When you're five foot six, there's nowhere to hide your weight. I put on a lot of weight, eating all the free hospital food, as you reminded me."

Karl shrugged.

"Your call, man. I'm cool with that. More for me."

"So what's up?"

"My pal Naunton Morgan just called me. He's on the medical executive committee at Abilene Memorial. He said they're discussing your application for consulting privileges *today*."

"Great!"

"So are you planning to leave Hotspur? Maybe move to Abilene?" Karl asked, hopefully. "I mean, I would support you one hundred percent. Or if you wanted to go somewhere else like Austin."

"Thank you. No, I'm not planning to leave. I've started doing more of my specialty work and I just wanted to have a safety net in case I had a complication."

"*Another* complication," Karl corrected.

"Yes, thank you. *Another* complication. Consulting privileges at Memorial allows you to directly admit up to two patients a year."

"You're sure you won't have more than two complications a year?" Karl asked, grinning widely.

"Karl, you know that was my first perforation. We've had this discussion before. Last night with Patty White I wished I had privileges at Memorial. I wouldn't have to beg Wegener or someone else to admit them. I could have admitted her directly to the ICU myself."

"What about taking call? If you have privileges at Memorial, they'll want you to take call there. How are you going to take call in Abilene if you live in Hotspur? We're sixty miles away."

"I read the rules and regulations of the hospital. If you take *consulting* privileges, you can only admit two patients a year but *you don't have to take call*."

Karl whistled.

"Now if you want *full* staff privileges, you have to take call," I continued.

Karl nodded.

"Man, that's perfect for you. But I'm worried. What if you perforate more than two patients a year?"

I glared at Karl.

"Then I will have to question everything I'm doing."

"If you get consulting privileges, can you consult on patients admitted by other doctors?"

"Yes."

"How many?"

"No limit," I smiled.

"Sweet! But of course no one is going to refer to you because they don't want to piss off Wegener. He can be pretty mean."

"I believe that. And I knew about the Medical Staff meeting in Abilene. It's at two p.m."

Karl held up a hand.

"Hold on. Are you going to attend it?"

"I'm going to try. I'm getting Patty transferred to Dallas Presbyterian. I've got to do that first."

"I figured you wanted to attend the Medical Staff meeting. That's why I wanted to tell you something. It's been moved up to ten am."

"What? No one told me! I can't get there at ten! I would have to leave by nine, in forty-five minutes!"

"The chief of staff called the meeting early. Guess who happens to be chief of staff?"

"Dr. Wegener?"

"Bingo! Naunton said he rearranged his surgery schedule to attend it and speak up for you. But he figured that Wegener had packed the meeting with his buddies and they were going to throw out your application."

"Throw it out? On what basis?"

Karl demolished a donut and took a long drag of coffee. He wiped his mouth with the back of his hand and stared at me dramatically.

"Tell me!" I repeated.

"You remember old Herschel Dunn from about a month ago?"

"Yes. The African-American man with bleeding from radiation damage to the rectum, aka radiation proctitis."

"You put him on formalin enemas."

"Yes. It stopped the bleeding,"

"I told you, formalin enemas were kind of weird. Can't say I didn't warn you."

"It's a standard treatment! It works!" I exclaimed.

"Did he get better?" Karl asked.

"I think so. He didn't come back for his follow-up appointment."

"He never does. Anyhow, he and his wife went shopping in Abilene and he became really sick and confused. So his wife took him to the ER at Memorial and Wegener was on call. They consulted him because of the history of rectal bleeding, even though he's not bleeding any more. Wegener got all bent out of shape on account of the formalin enemas and said that's what made Herschel toxic and confused."

"That's ridiculous! It doesn't do that!"

"Wegener did a CT scan and it showed some inflammation in the rectum, Einstein."

"But that could be due to the radiation proctitis itself! That's just the underlying disease that we're treating. Did he do a colonoscopy to check the lining?"

"No. He said it would be too dangerous."

"So he just claimed that the formalin enemas made Herschel toxic and sick but he didn't look at the rectal lining to see if the formalin had actually caused any harm!"

"Like I said, he said it was too risky. He just went with the CT scan."

"Unless you had done a CT scan before and after the formalin you can't say that the changes are due to the formalin! Radiation causes swelling of the rectum all the time! That's ridiculous!"

Karl nodded and spoke soothingly.

"I know, I know. So here's the bad part. Wegener wants to report you to the State Board. But he doesn't want to be the one accusing you. He wants the Medical Executive Committee to do his dirty work for him."

I reeled.

"This isn't bad, it's terrible! I can't believe I'm in so much trouble for a standard treatment."

"Just thought I'd give you a head's up and save you a trip to Abilene. Abilene might not be the right move for you right now."

I looked despondently at my cup. The coffee had cooled and I had lost my appetite.

"They're fixing to kick your ass out, Einstein."

"I'm going to ask that they put me on speaker phone," I said.

"Wow, that's gutsy. You want to be present at your own funeral?"

"Yes. Whom should I talk to?"

"Call the Memorial CEO, his name's Michael Morris. He's a good guy, a straight shooter. Tell him what's going on and he'll do his best. He may not be able to bend the rules for you but he'll see to it you get a fair trial and quick execution."

I winced.

"Thank you. Should I call the members of the Executive Committee?"

"Ask Michael Morris. But there's hardly any time and those attending will be Wegener's buddies. Save your breath."

Karl got up and walked to the door. He rubbed his hands.

"Call me if you're doing the speaker phone thing. I've got to hear this."

I stood up and left with him.

"I'm going to finalize Patty's transfer, then call Michael Morris," I said, grimly.

I had an incredible heaviness in the pit of my stomach. My mouth was dry and my hands were trembling. I felt terrible.

* * *

"Welcome to the Abilene Memorial Medical Executive Staff Committee. Thank you all for attending this special meeting. I'm Michael Morris and I'm the CEO of Abilene Memorial. Dr. Mathur, who is on the agenda, is with us via speakerphone. Can you hear us, Dr. Mathur?"

"Yes, I can, Mr. Morris. Thanks for allowing me to listen in and present my case."

There was an uncomfortable silence.

"You're welcome. Call me Mike. As you know, you're not on staff yet, but we're fixing to review your application for consulting privileges right now," Mr. Morris said.

Someone slapped the table.

"No! It's the fourth item on the agenda," Dr. Wegener snapped. "I don't know when we will get to it."

"But we have the doctor on speaker phone and I'm sure he's got patients to see," Michael said.

"Let's start with him," I heard Naunton Morgan growl.

"Who else is listening besides you?" Michael asked.

"Dr. Karl Becker is in the room with me. No one else."

"Okay. So I'm going to hand over to Dr. Wegener, our Chief of Staff."

I heard a microphone thud and screech as it was transferred, then the cold voice of Dr. Wegener.

"We have received and reviewed Dr. Mathur's application. However, serious charges have been brought against him. Patient injury, patient neglect, and patient endangerment. You can read the details in the hand-out in your folders. In summary, Dr. Mathur prescribed a highly toxic and controversial treatment for radiation proctitis to one of my patients. The bleeding had been controlled by conventional treatments that I had started. There was no reason to use this dangerous treatment. However, Dr. Mathur recklessly used formalin enemas to treat this patient and the patient developed severe sepsis and confusion. The details of the case and the labs and CT findings are also in your hand-outs."

There was a general rustling of papers as the doctors reviewed the records.

"Hey, Marty, why do we have to read this? We just got to vote on his application, right?" I heard someone say.

"These are serious failings. The motion before the Committee is to refer the matter to the State Board for urgent review," Dr. Wegener said.

Michael Morris coughed.

"Urging the State to review a doctor is tantamount to asking for an inquiry. This could put his license in jeopardy, please know that," he said, gravely.

"I have something to say," I said.

"You're not a member of our staff. You don't get to say anything," Dr. Wegener said, crisply.

"I'm sorry but you're sitting there passing judgment on me and setting up a meeting early without informing me and not even giving me the documents to review. That's not fair."

"What's not fair is that you want to work in this hospital and have admission privileges and see any number of consults and not take call! That's unfair!" Dr. Wegener replied.

"Okay, I'm going to intervene," Michael said. "I say we give Dr. Mathur a chance to present his case before deciding whether to refer him to the State Board."

"I decide that, I decide who speaks," Dr. Wegener said. "I'm the Chief of Medical Staff."

"Might be interesting to hear another point of view. Just for the sake of variety," Naunton drawled.

"He deserves a chance," Michael agreed. "And I'm having the patient's labs and CT faxed to his office right now so he can review the evidence against him."

"You mean, give him half a chance? Before his execution? That's a novel idea!" Naunton said, dryly.

There was silence. I jumped in.

"Thank you. I will be brief. Dr. Wegener and I have a common patient who is on Coumadin, a blood thinner, five milligrams daily. He had radiation treatment for prostate cancer and had been constantly losing blood from the rectum. He did respond briefly to local measures like steroids and laser coagulation but they stopped working. He became so anemic he needed a blood transfusion. We don't want to stop the blood thinner because there's a risk of stroke. So I tried formalin enemas. This treatment is not a dangerous treatment and is actually a well-accepted treatment," I said.

"It caused inflammation of the rectum! The rectum was all inflamed. Look at the CT!" Dr. Wegener snarled.

Tracy handed me the fax. I scanned the labs and CT report rapidly.

"Radiation proctitis itself can cause inflammation. Do you have CT scans before and after the formalin enemas were used?" I asked.

"No."

"So how do you know the formalin caused the swelling and not the radiation itself? How do you know the swelling wasn't *already* there before the formalin was used?"

"The patient became septic and confused after the formalin enemas were used!" Dr. Wegener crowed. "Explain that!"

"Mr. Dunn has difficulty passing urine. He has been using antihistamines and decongestants. I suspect he had urinary issues and a UTI. I suspect he had a urinary tract infection and that caused his confusion. The commonest reason for sudden confusion in the elderly is an infection."

"Let's look at the lab data. There's nothing about a urine test. Was one done?" Michael Morris asked.

Dr. Wegener hesitated.

"Yes, but I left it out because I didn't think it was relevant," he said. I rifled through the fax again.

"I don't have the urine report," I complained.

"No one does. It's not in the folder," Dr. Wegener answered.

"Why not?"

"It's not relevant."

I sensed hesitation in his voice. That gave me hope.

"Dr. Wegener, you have the complete medical record. Is there a urine report on Mr. Dunn?" I persisted.

No answer.

"Dr. Wegener, the urine report is critical. Do you have it?"

"It's not relevant."

"I think it is relevant. The commonest cause for confusion in the elderly is infection. Mr. Dunn has prostate problems. He could easily develop a urinary infection. That would explain the fever and confusion."

"I'm aware of the differential diagnosis of fever and confusion in the elderly. I don't need you to teach me basic medicine!"

"I'm trying to figure out what really happened. So what was the urine report?"

There was rustling.

"What do you want to know?"

"Just tell me if there were white cells in the urine."

"There were."

"How many?"

"Not sure. I would have to check."

"Please check."

"We don't have time! We have other matters! We have already wasted too much time in this ridiculous matter!"

Naunton coughed.

"*I* want to know. How many white cells in the urine?"

There was another pause.

"Fifty."

"What? *Fifty* white cells?"

"Did you not hear?"

"Fifty white cells per high power field?"

"Yes."

Naunton whistled.

"Well, I think that's pretty damn significant," he said.

"The urine report is not part of the official transcript of this meeting," Dr. Wegener said.

"Why not?"

"It was requested by someone who isn't a staff member. So it's not part of the official record."

"Dr. Wegener, Dr. Becker and I heard you and so did everyone in your meeting. It's on the record."

"We will have no record of the urine report."

"With fifty white cells per high power field, we all know that it's a urinary infection! Did the urine cultures grow anything?"

"I don't have that report back yet."

"Why not? It's been over a week. It doesn't take that long."

"Don't talk to me like that! I don't need to talk to you! I don't need to explain anything to you!"

"I'm just trying to defend myself and help the patient."

"Oh you are, are you? Such a good doctor? If you're such a good doctor, how come you couldn't make it in your own damn country?"

There was a shocked silence,

"I feel we get all the useless foreign doctors who weren't successful in their own countries, we get all the rejects," Dr. Wegener snapped. "And I'm not the only one who feels that way."

"Speak for yourself," Naunton growled.

I was furious.

"Let me tell you something. I'm Board certified. I have membership of the Royal College of Physicians of England. I'm board certified in internal medicine and gastroenterology, so I'm as qualified as you are!" I snapped.

"I was first in my graduating class at Yale. That means something. Everyone from India has a gold medal, sometimes five or ten gold medals. It's laughable. Those foreign qualifications mean nothing!"

"I must interrupt. Let's not get personal. Let's read the final report and decide what to do with Dr. Mathur's application," Michael Morris urged. Dr. Wegener went on.

"If he's such a wonderful doctor, how come he's in a tiny little town that no one has ever heard of? Why didn't he go back to India? He should go back to India."

I jumped in.

"Listen to me. Just like all of you, I'm looking for the best possible life for my family. I want to give them the best opportunities they could ever have. True, I had never heard of Hotspur or Abilene when I lived in London. We just came and fell in love with Texas. That's why we wanted to stay and not go back to London or India. I know I can be successful in London or India. We just like Texas and I want to give it a shot. But I'll tell you what I don't want. I don't want to be bullied around and be told where to go."

There was a rumbling.

"I'm still concerned about what Dr. Mathur did. I vote to send a letter of concern to the state board," Dr. Wegener said.

"Hold on," I said.

"Why? I've presented the case. Let's just vote on it now. Raise your hands if you're in agreement to send the letter."

There was a pause.

"Looks like the majority wants to send the letter," Michael sighed.

I stared at Karl in shock and dismay.

"No. I don't want to get into this mess. I'm sure Mr. Dunn was confused and sick because of the urinary infection. I know I will clear myself if you do report me. But I don't want to go through an investigation. How about if I withdraw my application for privileges?"

"You should have never applied!" Dr. Wegener gloated.

"I just wanted somewhere to put my patients in case they got sick or had a complication,"

"You shouldn't be practicing a specialty out in the sticks. You should just do family practice."

"But I'm a specialist! I've done thousands of procedures! I just want to have a little back-up, a safety net just in case."

"You serve no purpose doing endoscopy out there in the boonies. You should be sending all that work to us, not cherry-picking the good stuff and sending us all the crap!"

I swallowed.

"Look, I will withdraw my application if you drop everything. Is that a deal?"

There was a buzz as this was discussed. Karl looked surprised.

"You're throwing in the towel?" he wondered. I shook my head.

Dr. Wegener returned.

"Okay. Maybe."

"But I have one condition. I'm going to apply to the other hospital instead, at Abilene Baptist. I don't want you to do anything to jeopardize my application there."

"But if you're a bad doctor at Memorial then you're a bad doctor at Baptist. I'm on staff at both places, I can't cover up your mistakes," Dr. Wegener said.

My mouth was dry. I knew I had no chance with the medical committee at Memorial.

"I ask you to not send the letter to the state board," I repeated.

"Oh, but we must, Dr. Mathur, we must! It's our duty to protect our patients!" Dr. Wegener said.

I was desperate.

"The quality of mercy is not strained," I blurted.

There was a pause.

"Quoting Shakespeare won't help you," Dr. Wegener said.

There was a longer pause.

"Dr. Mathur? Are you there?"

"Yes."

"The medical executive committee just voted to send the matter to the State Board for review."

Dr. Wegener sounded triumphant.

"Can you take that back?" I asked.

"No. It's signed and sealed."

"I request you to reconsider. I will apply to Baptist instead."

"No. Too late."

"Are you reporting me as a committee or individually?"

"We are reporting you as a committee! I have the report written up and we are faxing it as we speak."

I was silent for a few minutes. Karl looked dazed. He shook his head slowly.

"Okay. Then I request that you ask the State Board for an expedited review. I am confident that they will find in my favor. I've reviewed the literature and formalin has never caused any confusion or sepsis. *Never.* Not once! I had the staff at the Texas Medical Association look it up for me. They will vouch for me. I also have a letter from my professors in Houston saying that formalin enemas are perfectly safe."

There was a rush of noise.

"I don't believe you," Dr. Wegener snarled.

"And I expect you to send me my privileges as soon as you hear back from Austin," I added.

"But we haven't even voted on that yet!"

"You just did. Your staff bylaws say that the medical executive committee may review the actions of any member of staff. But you don't have the power to investigate anyone who's *not* on your staff," I said.

"That's ridiculous! We have the right to report a bad doctor anytime!"

"You can report a bad doctor anytime as an *individual.* However, a medical executive committee can only censure it's own members. You don't have any authority. Read your own rules. It's right there."

There was stunned silence. Karl laughed out loud.

"So now that you've voted as a committee to have me reviewed, I have to be on staff. If you say I'm not on staff, then every one of you has exceeded your authority and the Texas Medical Association says that I can sue you all individually and the hospital as well. You don't obey your own rules."

There was a muffled discussion. I dug in deeper.

"Read your own bylaws. Page eight, paragraph three. It's all there."

"I don't believe this!" Dr. Wegener shouted. "What the *fuck?*"

I disconnected the phone.

"You set them up, didn't you, you little shit? I love it!" Karl guffawed. He jumped up and thumped my back.

"I had to be prepared. Naunton warned me. I figured, no one ever reads the rules. So I did. It's all right there. I just had to make sure they all voted on me as a committee. Once they did, it was over."

Karl shook his head slowly.

"You led them into it, didn't you? You knew what you were doing."

"I didn't know about the urinary infection."

"I bet that's the cause of his confusion."

"Far and away, the most likely cause. And formalin has never, ever been reported to cause an infection. So I feel good about that."

"Common things are common," Karl nodded.

"I just read the rules carefully."

"They never saw it coming," Karl grinned.

"You don't show up for a gunfight with a pocketknife."

Karl headed out the door.

"You fight like a Texan! How'd you figure all that out?" he laughed.

"I wasn't born in Texas, but got here as fast as I could," I said.

CHAPTER 18
THE WORST POSSIBLE DIAGNOSIS

"Thank you so much for seeing me, Dr. Mathur. I've been very upset."

"It's a pleasure to meet you, Mrs. Auzinger. You look familiar. Is this really your first visit to my clinic?"

"Yes, it is. At least, I think it is."

"I feel I've met you before."

"But I don't remember you, Doctor. Mind you, my daughter says I'm forgetting things. At least, I think my daughter says it. Maybe my son says it. Oh, I don't know!"

"Nevertheless, it's good to meet you. I see you're seventy-six years old, a retired elementary school teacher, widowed, and you live in Jasper. "

She nodded.

"Yes. That's right. And there was something else my daughter wanted me to tell you but I can't remember. I'm very upset. I can't remember what else she said, but I'm very upset. I've got something to tell you."

"Would you like me to call your daughter?"

"No. Let's go ahead."

"Tell me what's bothering you."

Mrs. Auzinger was a short, squat lady with shoulder-length hair dyed ferociously black. She wore thick rhinestone glasses, a sequined white shirt adorned with a green brooch that said *Noel*, and red slacks.

"I've been very upset. *Very* upset. Just after Easter, I went to see my regular doctor because I was hurting so much."

"It's almost two months since Easter now, so you mean you've been hurting for two months?"

"No, just about a month."

"Okay, so you've been hurting for a month. Where have you been hurting?"

"Everywhere. I lie down and my back hurts. I use the wrong pillow and my neck bothers me. I ate chili the other day and my gallbladder acted up. So I went to the Emergency Room."

"Did they find anything wrong?"

"Who?"

"The doctors in the ER, when you went to the Emergency Room?"

"I don't know. You'll have to ask my daughter. I was hurting too much to remember anything."

"Tell me more about the pain in your stomach."

"What about it? I've told you about it."

I was getting nowhere.

"Where, exactly, do you hurt? Which part of your abdomen hurts?" I asked.

"Well, sometimes it doesn't hurt. I don't know why it just stops."

Mrs. Auzinger shrugged helplessly

"But when it does hurt, where does it bother you?"

"Here and there. Everywhere."

"Where does it hurt the most?"

She pondered,

"In my neck, when I use a big pillow."

"No, I mean, where in your stomach area does it hurt the most?"

"Sometimes on the left and sometimes on the right."

"Which side hurts more often, the right side or the left?"

She paused.

"The right."

"Okay. Right upper or right lower part?"

"Here," she pointed.

"Okay, the right lower quadrant. Now, how long does it last?"

"Sometimes it lasts the whole day,"

"But how long does it *usually* last?"

"You mean, the pain?"

"Yes. How long does the pain usually last?"

She hesitated. I spoke up.

"Does the pain last a few seconds, a few minutes or an hour? Or more than an hour?"

"Sometimes an hour."

"Okay. Does anything make it worse?"

"Make it worse?"

"Like eating or bending or lying down, for instance. Or having a bowel movement. Do those things make the pain any worse?"

"No."

"Do they make the pain any better?"

"No."

"Does the pain wake you up at night?"

"Sometimes," she nodded.

"Sometimes? One night a month, or one night a week or several nights a week?"

"I don't know. I don't know. Maybe one or two nights a week."

"Wakes you out of your sleep?"

"Oh, yes! Yes, sir-ee!"

"Then what do you do, after it wakes you up from your sleep?"

"I get up and walk."

"Does that help?"

"Yes! Oh, my, it sure does!"

"Have you ever tried a heating pad?"

"Yes."

"Does it help?"

"Yes."

"A little or a lot?"

"It helps a lot."

"That's a helpful clue. Any fever or chills?"

"Sometimes I feel very warm. "

"But do you have a fever?"

"I think so. Maybe."

"Have you checked your temperature?"

"No."

"Any other medical problems, like heart disease or lung problems?"

"No."

"I'm looking at your list of medications. You're on thyroid hormones and medicine for high blood pressure. You're also taking a medicine called memantine for memory loss. Any other medicines or supplements?"

"No."

"You've had a hysterectomy and gall bladder surgery. Anything else?"

"I've had a colonoscopy. That's why I'm so upset."

"Why? Was there a problem with the colonoscopy?"

"Yes. The doctor missed a big cancer!" she wailed.

I paused.

"This is serious. Are you sure?"

"I got a CT scan done for the pain I was having. They did it in the ER. And they said, there's cancer in your colon. And I said, no, no, that's not possible. Because I just had a colonoscopy this year and it was clear."

I hesitated and asked the big question.

"Do you remember who did the colonoscopy?"

"Dr. Wegener. Dr. Wegener in Abilene."

I exhaled slowly. I started to feel a vicious energy.

"Are you sure?" I asked, cautiously.

"Of course I'm sure! I'm so mad at him! The CT scan showed there was a cancer in my colon and some spots on my liver! Stage four colon cancer! That's the worst possible diagnosis! I've got colon cancer and it's already spread to my liver!"

I was overwhelmed.

"I'm going to die because Dr. Wegener missed my colon cancer!" she cried.

"Mrs. Auzinger, you do have memory loss. Maybe you don't have all the facts."

"Why do you think I have memory loss?"

"You're wearing Christmas clothes in July. You're on memantine, a medicine for memory loss. So you may not have all the facts down perfectly."

She was irritated.

"I wish my daughter were here," she said.

I saw an envelope sticking out of her purse.

"Let me review the CT scan," I said.

I read the report.

"There is a soft tissue density in the cecum. This could be redundant tissue or a neoplasm. There is diverticular disease of the sigmoid colon. Additionally there are ill-defined lucencies in the liver. These could represent cysts or possibly secondary neoplasms. "

I tried to reassure her.

"It's not definite that there's cancer in the colon. It could be tissue that got folded up. Sometimes the lining of the colon gets folded up and on CT scans it looks like a growth."

"No, I just *know* it's cancer and it's causing my pain! I'm so upset! I just get up and pace around in my room. I just keep walking and bumping into things. That cancer should have been discovered by Dr. Wegener!"

Part of me was gleeful.

"Dr. Wegener missed the cancer! And now it's spread!" she lamented. "And I'm going to die because of his mistake!"

I wondered what to say. I was delighted at the prospect of revenge. I hated Dr. Wegener and this opportunity had just fallen into my lap. I was surprised at what I said next.

"Well, we just need to repeat the colonoscopy and find out whether there really is a cancer there or not. It's possible that it's just a fold. Maybe he didn't make a mistake."

Mrs. Auzinger was doubtful.

"Would a fold make me hurt?" she asked.

"No," I admitted.

"See? I knew it, there's a big bad cancer sitting there. And Dr. Wegener missed it! How could he miss it?"

"It's not certain that it's a cancer. And yes, it's possible to miss a cancer on colonoscopy. In the cecum, the lower right part of the colon where the CT sees something, there's a valve and sometimes a polyp can be hidden behind that valve."

"So it's okay to miss a polyp or cancer?"

"No, I'm just saying that colonoscopy is not a hundred percent effective all the time. Sometimes we miss things."

"Isn't Dr. Wegener a famous specialist?"

"Yes. He's very good."

"Did you know he was top of his class in Yale?"

I choked a little.

"Then how come he missed my cancer?"

"Let's not jump to conclusions, Mrs. Auzinger."

Mrs. Auzinger was irate.

"But isn't it a big deal to miss cancer?"

I hesitated. I wanted to skewer Wegener myself, but I held back.

"It's possible to miss polyps or small cancers," I admitted.

"So could *you* have missed it?"

I thought about it.

"It's possible. Yes."

She scowled.

"But I'm still mad at him. I don't know what to do. Stage four! I'll be dead in a few months. His mistake is going to cost me my life!"

Abruptly, there was a knock on the door. It was flung open and a young lady marched in. She was tall, had short black hair, designer glasses and purple lipstick. She sported a black handbag with gold chains and surveyed the room. She quickly perched on the chair next to Mrs. Auzinger and placed her handbag in the floor. There was a strong smell of lavender perfume.

"I'm Shelly Morganthal, her daughter," she said and extended her hand. We shook warmly.

"Nice to meet you," I said.

"Don't you remember me?" she asked.

"Not really," I admitted.

"We saw you in Houston, before you left for Hotspur. Mother was your patient in Houston."

I gazed at Mrs. Auzinger again.

"That's why she seemed so familiar. But she denied it," I said.

Shelly smiled indulgently at her mother.

"Mother doesn't remember things. She has a touch of Alzheimer's. But you were her gastroenterologist in Houston."

I suddenly felt a sense of dread.

"*You're* the one who did her colonoscopy some years ago," she declared.

"No, honey, it was Dr. Wegener," Mrs. Auzinger said.

"No, Mother. Dr. Wegener did an upper scope for you in February. It was normal. But it was Dr. Mathur who did your colonoscopy. He did it in Houston one or two years ago. When I heard he was practicing in Hotspur, I thought, great, we can go back to him. I've got a copy of your report."

I felt terrible. She pulled out a folded paper from her handbag. I read it with dismay. Mrs. Auzinger gazed at me with astonishment.

"So *you* were the one who did my colonoscopy?" she asked.

I read the report again.

"Yes, I was the one," I admitted

"So *you* missed my cancer!"

"Well, I certainly hope not. I don't know. I'm not sure. All I can say is, we really need to do another colonoscopy right away to find out."

Mrs. Auzinger pushed her chair back and crossed her arms.

"I'm very upset. There are spots on my liver, and the ER doctor said that means the cancer has spread to my liver! Did I tell you that?"

"Yes, you did. That would be very bad. But there's a chance those spots are just little cysts."

"What are cysts?"

"Collections of clear fluid. Cysts are not cancer."

"Do you think the spots on my liver are cysts?"

"Possibly."

"You're not sure?"

"No. But let's not get diverted. Let's set up the colonoscopy."

"Where will we do it?"

"Well, I recently got consulting privileges at Abilene Memorial. You live near Abilene so that would be convenient for you."

Mrs. Auzinger looked at her daughter. Shelly nodded.

"Let's set it up. I want it done as quickly as possible. I can't rest. I've been pacing up and down all over my house, I'm so nervous. I'm so upset, so upset."

I felt hollow and worthless. I pulled myself together.

"Let me explain how to get ready for this test," I said, trying to sound normal.

I explained the process to both of them and gave them the instructions. We went to the checkout window. Mrs. Auzinger grasped my wrist.

"I still can't believe you missed my cancer," she complained. "Do you know it's stage four?"

It was one of the worst evenings ever. I tried to remember details of the colonoscopy I had done for Mrs. Auzinger, but I had no specific memory of that procedure. Had I been rushed? Had I withdrawn the scope too fast? Had the clean-out been poor? That could have obscured my vision. I imagined missing a large cancer and I wondered if Mrs. Auzinger would sue me or forgive me.

I remembered feeling gleeful and superior, when I thought that Dr. Wegener had done the procedure, and the crushing realization as I read my own report. I imagined what the other doctors and nurses would say.

I remembered one of Penny's sayings: *when you point a finger at someone, there are three pointing back at you.*

CHAPTER 19

THE BIG REVEAL

Three days later we were in the gastroenterology suite at Abilene Memorial. Mrs. Auzinger was lying on her left side on the endoscopy table. Her daughter, Shelly, stood near her head and held her hand. Mrs. Auzinger was uncomfortable and rocked back and forth. She complained to her daughter. The nurse, Greg Nazier, had started an IV. Andy Babineaux, the anesthetist, had drawn up two syringes of propofol and was ready. There was another lady standing in the room. I did not recognize her, so I went to her.

"Good morning. I'm Dr. Mathur. I don't believe we've met," I said.

"Good morning, Doctor. I'm Lyssa Saverance. I'm the Physician Coordinator and I'm from Administration."

She was a short, plump lady with high blonde hair and bangs. She smiled excessively.

"What are you doing here in the GI lab?" I asked.

"I was there when you had the phone interview with the medical executive committee. Dr. Wegener asked me to observe your endoscopy to make sure your skills were acceptable."

I was angry.

"I'm board certified! I've completed a fellowship at Baylor, and I've also trained in London. I've done over two thousand colonoscopies!"

"And you had one perforation. Therefore there is a quality concern," she beamed.

"Do you do this kind of observation routinely?"

Lyssa hesitated, then smiled broadly.

"No."

"So am I getting special attention?"

"Just a matter of quality, doctor."

"Is this routine?" I persisted.

"I'm just here to observe," Lyssa said, baring her teeth tightly.

Shelly Morganthal broke in.

"Excuse me. My mother has a problem, she's upset," she said.

I returned to Mrs. Auzinger.

"Good morning, Mrs. Auzinger. I know you're hungry and thirsty. We will get started in just a minute," I said.

"That's not the problem. Doctor, I was pacing in my bedroom and my big toe hit the side of an old chair. I've got a wood splinter under my nail, in my big toe! It's *killing* me!"

I examined her foot. There was a sliver of wood jammed like a dagger under the first right toenail. A crimson streak of coagulated blood had developed around the splinter like a sheath and had lifted the nail up. I ran my finger gently under the nail's edge. Mrs. Auzinger shuddered. The splinter had broken off under the nail and there was nothing projecting out. I touched the surface of the nail and she jumped.

"Ow! That's really painful!" she cried.

"I'm sorry, but it's totally underneath your toenail. It's going to be difficult to get it out."

"Please get it out. It's really hurting!"

"It does look painful. But we need to do the colonoscopy and then I can send you to the ER to have that splinter taken out."

Mrs. Auzinger shook her head adamantly.

"Oh, no. No, no! That thing is hurting like a son of a gun! I want that fixed! I'm not doing the colonoscopy until you get that out!"

I was in a quandary. Lyssa watched me curiously.

"How about this: let's do the colonoscopy and then I will personally take you to the ER?" I offered.

"No," Mrs. Auzinger said, resolutely. "I want you to get the splinter out first."

"Would you like me to numb it up your toe, then do the colonoscopy?"

"No, I want you to take the darn thing out first!"

I gazed at her, confused.

"I'm not going ahead with the colonoscopy unless you fix my toe! Period!" Mrs. Auzinger thundered.

I knew I had to address the toe. I sent Greg to the ER to pick up a minor surgery kit.

"Okay, Mrs. Auzinger, I'm going to try to remove the splinter. I've sent the nurse down to get me some numbing medicine and a fine-tipped forceps. I'm going to numb up your toe, then cut a little wedge out of the top of your nail so I can get to the splinter. I'll have to cut through the sensitive area."

"Do whatever you have to do! It's sore as a raisin! I need help!"

She grasped her daughter's hand and moaned.

"So how are you going to explain the charges for the kit from the ER?" Lyssa asked.

"What do you mean?"

"Well, your patient is here for colonoscopy. How are you going to explain why you worked on her toe?"

"I'm going to write a detailed addendum and explain exactly what happened. The patient was in distress so I'm going to help her. That's what we're *supposed* to do, right? Help our patients?"

"Who will pay for the medicines and equipment to remove the splinter?"

"I've done these before in Hotspur. There's a code for it and I can bill Medicare. It's a standard code."

Lyssa was not impressed.

"You will have to document it properly. I don't think you can do a colonoscopy and add *removal of a splinter from the big toe.*"

"No, they are two separate and distinct procedures."

"You don't have hospital privileges for splinter removal."

"That's ridiculous. I'm a specialist and that means I've done all the basic requirements of a generalist. You can't be a specialist without being a general internist. If you've given me specialist privileges, general privileges are understood."

"I need to check this with Administration."

"Go ahead. Ask Michael Morris."

Lyssa disappeared into a dictation room to make the call. Greg returned with the kit. We turned Mrs. Auzinger onto her back and I cleaned the right foot with iodine and alcohol. I draped the foot with clean towels, leaving only the big toe exposed. I put on gloves, mask and gown.

"Mrs. Auzinger, I'm going to inject lidocaine into the sides of your big toe. It's going to hurt."

She yelped as I injected dilute lidocaine into both sides of the toe.

"What are you using, Doctor?" Lyssa asked.

"Lidocaine," I replied.

"Is it lidocaine with epinephrine, or just plain lidocaine?"

I paused and stared at her.

"Lidocaine *without* epinephrine. We both know that epinephrine is harmful during this kind of nerve block."

Lyssa smiled and nodded.

"You're asking questions and setting a trap," I said.

Lyssa shrugged and looked away. I turned back to Mrs. Auzinger.

"Now the toe will be numb. I'm going to cut into the top of your nail and make a little notch."

"I don't feel anything now, Doctor."

"Good. I'm cutting your nail with a sharp tipped forceps. I'm trying to get to the upper end of the splinter."

"Then what?"

"Okay, I've made a pretty big notch. Now I'm going to have Greg push up on your toenail so the splinter doesn't slip down any more."

I strapped on magnifying lenses.

"I can see the top of the splinter. There's a little bleeding from where I cut the notch, that's interfering with finding the splinter."

Greg pulled on sterile gloves and gripped the base of the toe with both thumbs. He pushed the splinter upwards. Mrs. Auzinger cried out.

"Hold still! I'm having a hard time grasping the top of the splinter!"

Mrs. Auzinger squirmed and Greg lost his grip. I lost the splinter.

"Okay, let's elevate the foot. That will reduce blood flow and engorgement. Then we can try again."

We elevated her foot and swabbed the toe. I used the magnifying glasses to find the jagged top of the splinter. I opened the forceps a fraction and slid the tips well past the top of the splinter into the fleshy pulp of the toe. Mrs. Auzinger gasped in pain

"I'm trying to get a good grip on the splinter!" Greg cried.

Mrs. Auzinger gasped again. I briefly thought about injecting some more lidocaine to improve the numbing, but I didn't want to lose my opportunity.

I gripped hard and wiggled the splinter. I was able to loosen it. Mrs. Auzinger started crying. Her daughter stepped in.

"Please, give her a break," she requested.

I waited a minute, but didn't let go of the splinter.

"Okay, I'm going to wriggle it again and then pull it. Are you ready?"

Mrs. Auzinger wiped her eyes and nodded.

I gripped the splinter and tugged but it wouldn't budge. I rotated it gingerly, worried it would snap. I untwisted and urged Greg to apply more pressure.

"I'm pressing really hard, Dr. Mathur!" he protested.

"More pressure!"

"Any more pressure and I might take her toe off!" Greg declared.

He squeezed with all his might. The toe turned dusky.

"Try now, Doc," he said.

"If you break the piece you'll have to pull the whole dang nail off," Andy, the anesthetist, warned.

I imagined the angle at which the splinter had entered. I turned a little so that I was pulling up and out, following the same imaginary line. I twisted and pushed in and then pulled out. I kept going back and forth until I could feel it loosen. I pulled out with sustained pressure.

"Okay, I'm pulling it out now!"

I pulled hard, but it wouldn't budge.

"Hurry up, Doc! We need to start the colonoscopy!" Andy said.

"It's not moving," I said.

"What do you mean?"

"It's stuck inside and I can't get it out!"

"That's what the bishop said to the actress," Andy cackled.

Lyssa gasped.

"That's completely inappropriate," she said. "Don't ever make those crude jokes again!"

Andy grinned widely.

I pulled harder. The splinter broke.

"Doc, she's hurting too much. I'm going to give her a little morphine," Andy said.

"Go ahead. Then I'm going to extend the notch on her nail and reach down into the pulp of the nail with the forceps."

Shelly, her daughter, shuddered.

"Just the thought of someone ripping up my nail and poking around inside my toe makes me really queasy," she said.

"I'm sorry, this sounds gory," I said.

"Do it, just do it," Shelly said, but withdrew a step and covered her eyes.

"Yo, Doc, hurry up! We haven't even started the darn scope yet!" Andy said.

I injected more lidocaine, cut a deeper notch, and slowly advanced the closed tips of the forceps. I felt the tips touch the stump.

"I'm opening up the tips and pushing down, this is going to hurt!"

But I couldn't separate the tips of the forceps.

"I'm going to cut the nail a little more," I warned.

Mrs. Auzinger cried out in apprehension. She tried to sit up. Greg held her shoulders down. Shelly covered her face and turned away.

"What a mess!" Lyssa said. I ignored her.

"Now the nail has a big V-shaped cut and I'm going to go deep and force the forceps open and grab the stump of the splinter. The splinter went deep inside your toe and broke, that's why it's so difficult to get it out. Greg, grab the base of the toe again. Give me a little force!"

Greg gripped the toe again. Mrs. Auzinger moaned.

I opened the tips of the forceps and closed them on the top of the stump. I squeezed tightly and pulled up and out with force. The stump shuddered, then suddenly shot out.

Mrs. Auzinger sat up and screamed. She lunged for her foot, and froze in mid-air. She opened her mouth to scream again.

"Doctor! What are you doing?" Lyssa cried.

"How does that feel, Mrs. Auzinger?" I asked.

Mrs. Auzinger stopped mid-scream. She froze for a few seconds, then smiled.

"Oh, that feels so good! *So good!* I can tell it's totally gone! Oh, thank you, thank you so much!"

I gazed at the splinter and the stump. Together, they were half an inch long and stippled with blood and strands of fat and fibrous tissue.

"Oh, that looks evil!" Shelly declared.

Andy coughed theatrically.

"Can we start now? I've got other patients that I need to put to sleep," he said.

I threw the splinter in the trash and cleaned up quickly.

"So how are you going to account for this little adventure?" Lyssa asked.

"I'm going to use the CPT code. I'm going to go strictly by the book.

I will write a note, and I will explain the indications and put in a full description."

Lyssa was not satisfied.

"You did an unnecessary procedure and will charge the hospital for it. How can we bill for it? What if her insurance doesn't pay? That's a loss for the hospital and a waste of resources," she said.

"No, we did a necessary medical service. Our patient was suffering. I did perform an unrelated procedure but it was medically necessary. And only a doctor decides if a procedure was necessary, not an administrator."

"How do you know she has Medicare?"

"Look at the screen. See her date of birth? She's in her seventies, so she has Medicare as her primary insurance and Medicare doesn't require precertification for these procedures. So the hospital will get paid."

"Was it a necessary procedure?"

"Of course. Did you not hear a thing she said? She was crying out in pain. And you question whether it's necessary? Remember, only the doctor decides if a procedure is necessary."

"Really? Who says that?" Lyssa demanded

"Your own policies and procedures manual. I read it carefully before the Executive Committee meeting."

Lyssa looked upset. I pushed my advantage.

"Also, you cannot stay in the room when I do the procedure. The patient has not given you her consent."

"I can ask her right now."

"No, you can't."

"Why not?"

"Because Andy already started the propofol."

"I can still ask her. She's not fully asleep yet."

"You can't take a consent once the anesthetic has started, even if they're awake. That's another rule."

Lyssa scowled.

"I'm going to ask you to step outside the room," Greg said and waved her outside. Shelly had already stepped out. After Lyssa left, we had Mrs. Auzinger lie on her left side. We turned the lights down. Andy sedated her completely and we finally began the colonoscopy.

"I bet you're nervous," Andy said.

"A little," I admitted.

"Just a little? You might have missed a cancer!"

"How do you know that?"

"Oh, I read the chart. Why do you think Lyssa is waiting? She's Dr. Wegener's stooge. She's here to nail you."

"*If* there's a cancer."

"Where are you now?"

"I'm the sigmoid colon."

"What's taking so long?"

"Her clean-out isn't good."

"Why is that?"

"She has dementia. She may not have understood the directions or followed them properly."

"Man, you're literally up shit's creek without a paddle," Andy grinned.

I washed and suctioned the colon lining and progressed slowly. I finally entered the very last part of the colon, the cecum. I looked around and slumped with relief.

"It's clear," I gasped.

I washed the cecum by injecting water. I stretched it open with gas and turned the tip of the scope backwards to make sure I hadn't missed anything.

"You can breathe again, Doc! Bet your ass sphincter was tight as a knot!" Andy chuckled.

I withdrew the scope gently. I looked around the colon carefully, washing and suctioning and pushing in gas to stretch it open.

"You still got to deal with Lyssa outside, Doc. You know where that name comes from?" Andy asked.

"No."

"Lyssa was the Greek goddess of rage. Kind of appropriate, right?"

I nodded.

"First. I'm going to talk to her daughter, Shelly. Then I'll deal with Lyssa," I said.

"So there was no cancer?" Lyssa asked.

"No,"

She looked disappointed

"A polyp?"

"No."

"Something wrong with the lining?"

"No. It was totally normal."

"Then why did the CT report say there was a growth?"

"It was just a fold."

"And the liver spots?"

"Just simple cysts, most likely."

"How can you be sure?"

"I found an old CT report on her liver from four years ago. The same liver spots were there four years ago and haven't changed in size or number."

Lyssa sighed.

"Okay. So how are you going to document removing the splinter?" she inquired.

"I'm going to add it to my colonoscopy note."

"How can you do that? That's not acceptable."

"I think her insurance will permit it, there's a clause that covers it," I smiled.

"Really? How?" Lyssa sneered. She got up to leave.

"Her insurance clearly says I can add a footnote."

I returned to my patient.

CHAPTER 20
WILDERNESS IS PARADISE NOW

Agatha and Tommy Templar sat on one side of our dining table. Priya and Anjali sat across from them, and Maya and I sat at the ends. I had opened a bottle of wine and Maya had just laid out dinner. She glanced at Tommy.

"Tommy, would you like to say a prayer?" she asked.

"Yes, I would. Let's hold hands and bow our heads. Heavenly Father, we ask that You bless this food. We ask that You help us use Your many gifts to strengthen us and do Your work. Bless the Mathurs as they work in the home and the school and the hospital. Accept our thanks for the rain and the fine wheat and cotton, and the other blessings You continue to bestow upon us in this part of Paradise. We say this in Christ's name. Amen."

Tommy looked up and smiled.

"Let's eat! It all looks delicious," he said.

"Maya, tell us about the food," Agatha said.

"The main dish is lamb biryani. That's soft cooked spicy lamb in rice, and I have some whipped yogurt next to it in case you feel it's too sharp. The third dish is potatoes and cauliflower, slow cooked with ginger and turmeric. It's really very simple."

"It looks and smells fabulous," Agatha said.

"I love biryani, and you have it with yogurt," Priya said. Anjali nodded.

"Tell us about biryani," Tommy said, as he helped himself.

"It's a Moghul dish. It was invented by the Moghuls when they invaded India. They rode all day on horseback and ate just once a day, so their cooks wanted to make a quick meal that was filling and gave them everything they needed," Maya said.

"A dish to fight over," Agatha said. "Tell us how you make it."

Maya nodded.

"I fry onions in butter and then add rice and water. I leave it on low heat for at least an hour. I cook the lamb separately, and add it later. I also brown some slivered onions and cashew nuts and golden raisins and add them just before serving," she said.

"It's amazing," Tommy said. "Normally, I don't like lamb, but this is just amazing!"

"It's delicious," Agatha agreed.

"Presh, does it hurt to eat?" Tommy asked. Agatha was embarrassed.

"No, not at all," she said. "What's that? Cauliflower? I'd like to try that."

I passed her the dish.

"I like potatoes and cauliflower as well, and it's not spicy," I said. "It's softer than the lamb," Tommy said.

Agatha took a spoonful.

"I'm not surprised to see potatoes. I think potatoes are in every cuisine. Were potatoes and peppers and spices all discovered in India?" she asked.

"Actually, presh, peppers originated in South America. I'm surprised I hadn't told you that before. They were taken by the Spanish back to Europe but the climate did not work. But the plants made their way to India, thanks to European explorers like Vasco da Gama. Peppers grew very well there."

"Actually, I do remember now. You did tell me that peppers and potatoes originated in South America. I am surprised I forgot. I think I've been distracted lately," Agatha said.

"I love potatoes," Anjali chirped. Tommy speared a potato with his fork and held it up.

"Behold the potato! The humble potato also came from the Andes. The Spanish took it back to Europe, and it changed the world," Tommy said.

"How did that happen?" Priya asked.

"Well, until then, Europe was dependent on wheat. But wheat was hard to grow and sometimes there would be very poor harvests, so Europe was always facing shortages of food and starvation and famine. But potatoes were easier to grow and more reliable. So suddenly Europe had enough to eat. Because of that, they were able to do great things in art and design and explore the world. The whole world changed forever."

Anjali swallowed a mouthful.

"The Renaissance was possible because of the potato," Tommy said.

"I like Mommy's potatoes," she repeated. Maya smiled.

"We all like your mother's cooking," Tommy nodded.

I served the wine and Tommy sipped it slowly.

"I see you're serving another Riesling, Sandy," he said.

"Yes, it's a sweet wine and robust enough to go with Indian food. I know you recognize the shape of the bottle."

"The wine is supposed to have a characteristic smell," Tommy said. He swirled the wine and sniffed it.

"Darling, it's not a smell, it's a bouquet," Agatha pointed out.

"Correct, I stand corrected. Riesling has a special kind of bouquet, but I can't quite describe it."

"It's supposed to smell a little like diesel," I said.

"Diesel? That doesn't sound right," Maya said.

"It smells faintly of diesel. Sauvignon blanc wines smell of grass. Those are two distinctive bouquets of wine."

"I like the way you've made the potatoes and cauliflower. What gives them the yellow color?" Agatha asked. "Saffron?"

"I put in a little turmeric. I also use roasted cumin and I leave the potatoes and cauliflower covered loosely on low heat for about thirty minutes."

"You must write that down for me. Our children live in DC and they rave about Indian food. They are just so tickled that we're eating this wonderful Indian meal here in Hotspur!"

We ate happily and talked about food and travel. The Templars told us about their children and grandchildren, all of whom lived in Washington, DC. They loved the city's museums and restaurants but were always plagued by traffic delays. Washington seemed a world away from us. We told them about growing up in India. We stayed at the table, and everyone had second helpings. Maya beamed at the six clean plates. Priya, Anjali, and I cleared the table and set out small plates. I started a pot of decaffeinated coffee.

"We have a special dessert for you to try, but I bought apple pie as back-up, just in case," Maya announced.

"Oh? What is it?" Agatha asked.

"It's a special dessert called carrot halwah. It's like a carrot brownie, or carrot cookie dough."

Agatha and Tommy exchanged glances.

"It sounds interesting. I'm in!" Agatha said.

"Maya, if you've made it, it must be good. I'm going to pass on the pie. I want your carrot dessert," Tommy agreed.

Maya served the halwah in two-inch squares, gleaming orange with white streaks, topped with pistachios and golden raisins. Agatha and Tommy ate cautiously.

"This is different," Tommy said. "I don't think I've ever eaten anything quite like this. It does taste like cookie dough. What do you think, presh?"

"I think it's like a sweet version of carrot salad, you know, with added nuts, and a creamy richness," Agatha said.

"You're right. It's a reduction of shredded carrots in milk and sugar. The concentrated milk gives it richness."

"No spices?" Tommy asked, smiling.

"None at all," Maya laughed.

The girls picked up the dessert plates and excused themselves. I poured coffee.

"I enjoyed hearing about the spices you used, and where they originated," Agatha said. "I'm surprised I had forgotten that Tommy had told me all about them. It's fascinating!"

"Tommy knows a lot. He told me about the distinctive bottles that are used for Rieslings."

"Oh, Tommy knows a lot. Sometimes the children would hesitate to ask him and complain, we don't want to know *that* much about everything."

"I'd like to read about the spices of the world," Tommy said.

"If I ever wrote about them, I would call it, 'Origin Of The Spices'," I chuckled.

"Except that Mr. Darwin is not always a popular figure in Hotspur," Tommy said.

"You remember Mark and Amanda Hastings?" Agatha asked. "We sent Mark to you when Amanda didn't want to see Dr. Becker."

"Yes, I remember. I got into a lot of trouble with Dr. Becker over that. She used to be his patient. *He* wanted to look after Amanda. He was upset and said I was stealing his prized patient."

"Yes, we heard all about it. Amanda also told us that you talked about evolution, and that the IV fluids you were using resembled sea water, and that we might have common ancestry with fish and amphibians and other animals."

"True. That's the basis of evolution."

"But not everyone in Hotspur believes in evolution. Some believe in Creationism, that God created us directly."

"What do you think?"

"I think - we think - that evolution is correct. We don't believe that it contradicts the Bible. But we know many others who disagree."

"What do the Hastings believe?"

"Creationism. They're passionate about it! Yet they really liked you, and have been talking you up all over town. They've sent you many patients."

"Even though they didn't like my views on evolution?"

"You took care of Amanda so well that they glossed over their differences and have become strong supporters."

"I'm surprised and grateful."

"God moves in strange and wondrous ways, His miracles to perform," Tommy smiled.

Agatha looked around.

"Your girls have gone to bed, and the two of you must be tired. We should be getting home," she said.

"Hold on, presh. We have an important message to convey to Sandy and Maya," Tommy said. Agatha nodded.

"Do forgive me. My mind wanders, I have not been able to focus. We do have a message for you from the hospital board," she said. "May I be very direct?"

I looked at Maya. We shrugged.

"The hospital board wants you to stay in Hotspur. We know that you are about to complete your three-year contract. You have made many positive changes in our little hospital. We are back in the black. We have paid off our debts. We have given our nurses a small raise for the first time in six years. Patients are coming back to the hospital and there is a confidence and trust that wasn't there before," Agatha said.

"And we feel that you deserve a good bit of credit," Tommy said. "So we really want you to stay. We want to renew your contract. What do you say?"

I was taken aback.

"That's very nice of you," I said. "I don't know what to say."

"We know that you have applied for jobs in Austin and Abilene, and you've obtained admitting privileges at Abilene Memorial Hospital. But you have such a strong base here, and the people here love you. Why go to a big city where nobody knows you? Why not stay here?" Tommy said.

I hesitated.

"I'm a specialist," I explained. "I do like practicing general medicine. But I really like being a specialist in gastroenterology."

"Are you not comfortable practicing general medicine?"

"I am comfortable. I enjoy it. I'm pretty confident in general medicine. But I was trained in gastroenterology, and I like doing procedures. We can stop someone's bleeding, remove a growth, stretch open a narrowed area, or do something you can't do with medicine alone."

"Can't you practice your specialty here in Hotspur?" Tommy asked.

"There aren't that many people in Hotspur. The town has only five thousand and the county has another five thousand. That's enough for general practice but not enough for a specialist."

"You talked about going to Bavaria and Winters and other small towns? You could do specialty clinics there, too. The people there would appreciate having a specialist come to their town. That would give you a large base."

"Those hospitals don't have the endoscopes and the equipment I need to do procedures."

Tommy leaned forwards and spoke slowly.

"How about if we let you take the equipment from Hotspur with you?" he said.

"How would I do that?"

"Our hospital has a van. Your equipment is on carts with wheels. We can build a ramp and just roll your towers into the van, and then strap them down. The van can follow you to Bavaria and other small towns."

"But how would you get paid for letting other hospitals borrow your scopes?"

"The hospitals charge the patient's insurance a facility fee, as you know. We would split the facility fee with them. So it's a win-win situation. The other hospital gets to do procedures in their OR, they get reimbursed, and then we get reimbursed as well. Everyone's happy."

"So I could do procedures in Bavaria and Winters? Even Colorado City?"

"You bet," Tommy grinned.

"How about Abilene? Could I take the equipment from Hotspur to a surgery center in Abilene?"

"Fine by me. I'm sure the board would actually be tickled. A specialist and specialty instruments going from little Hotspur to big old Abilene! I love it!"

I looked at Maya.

"Well, that would give me plenty of specialty work to do. I could do gastroenterology clinics in Bavaria and Winters and Colorado City and Abilene, but keep Hotspur as my base!"

"Exactly! So what do you think?"

"I'm interested. But I need a little more time to discuss this with Maya and think this through."

"Sure. Think about it as much as you like, but we would like to have your decision within a couple or three days."

"Two or three days? That's all?"

"If you leave, we would have to start looking for your replacement right away. It takes time."

"I understand. I will let you know soon."

"We hope we don't have to look for a replacement," Tommy said.

Tommy and Agatha pushed back from the table. We all got up.

"What a delightful evening," Agatha said. "We enjoyed it so much!"

"And to think we almost didn't make it!" Tommy added.

"What do you mean?" Maya asked.

"Agatha was having a terrible headache all morning and afternoon. She's been having them for months, off and on. We were thinking about canceling but Agatha insisted that she was better."

That caught my attention.

"Hold on. It was a severe headache? Really painful?" I asked.

Agatha paused.

"Why did you have to bring that up, presh?" she chided Tommy. "Let's just go home. I can see a doctor tomorrow."

"You were really in agony, dearest. You've been a little disoriented and forgetful all day. You said the pain was so bad you couldn't see properly!"

I interrupted.

"Wait! Stop a moment. Did you lose vision?"

"Yes, but just for an hour or so. It came back."

"Put down your jackets and sit down. This could be serious," I said.

"It's just a bad headache," Agatha said. "We'll sort it out later."

"Any other problems?"

"No."

"Are you sure?"

"Yes."

"Did your face or arms or legs go weak?"

"The right side of my head felt very sensitive. Could barely comb my hair on that side."

"Which side was the headache?" I persisted.

"The right side."

"Okay. How long did it last?"

"At least eight hours. Maybe more."

"And it caused blurred vision?"

"Yes."

"Any pain in the jaw muscles, after you have finished brushing and flossing?"

"I'm surprised that you ask. I haven't understood why, but sometimes I do get severe pain from chewing food. Especially bread and meat."

"So that's why Tommy was asking you if you were able to eat the lamb, and saying that the cauliflower was softer."

"Yes. Sometimes my jaw muscles hurt so much when I eat that I simply give up and skip the meal."

"That's significant. I thought that maybe the lamb was too tough for you."

"Oh no, the lamb was to die for! It was fall-off-the-bone tender! It didn't hurt me."

Maya was reassured. I leaned forwards.

"This is important. Do your jaw muscles hurt before, during or after eating?" I asked.

"They hurt during and after eating."

"Never before?"

"No. Why do you ask?"

"Because that means that the blood supply to your jaw muscles is sufficient at rest, but not sufficient when the muscles are active. That means a partial blockage of the blood supply to those muscles."

"That makes sense."

"Does the pain become severe?"

"No, but it scares me. I'm afraid to eat because I don't want it to hurt more. So I've been eating less."

"How's your weight?"

"I've lost five pounds in the last couple of months."

"I don't like the sound of this. Please sit down again, both of you. Agatha, I'm going to examine you. I'm going to get my flashlight and knee hammer from my car."

Agatha and Tommy looked uncomfortable. Priya and Anjali reappeared in the doorway in their pajamas and watched curiously, swinging in and out of the doorframe. Maya sat down next to Agatha and held her hand.

"I think he just wants to check you, just to be safe," she said.

Agatha nodded numbly. I returned and sat next to her.

"Agatha, I'm going to shine this light in your eyes. I'm going to see how your pupils respond."

"Go ahead."

"Now look at the tip of my finger and focus on it as I bring it close to your face."

Her pupils responded properly.

"Now let me touch both sides of your face. Does it feel the same on both sides? "

"It actually feels more sensitive on the right side."

I palpated the artery on the right temple. Agatha flinched. The artery on the left was not tender at all.

"I'm going to do a brief neurological exam, Agatha. Raise your eyebrows, please. Now smile, show me your teeth. Good! Open your mouth and stick out your tongue and move it from side to side. Now put your tongue back in your mouth and say *ahh*."

"Is everything okay?" Tommy interrupted.

"Yes. Agatha, shrug your shoulders. Now turn your head from one side to the other."

She complied readily.

"Now I'm going to test your reflexes in your arms and legs. Then I'm going to test sensation in your arms and legs."

I checked her knee and elbow reflexes and touched corresponding sites in her arms and legs, using the base of the knee hammer.

"It feels the same on both sides."

"Good. Your reflexes are normal as well."

"So what have you found?"

I took a deep breath.

"Your exam is normal except for tenderness over your right temple and the artery in that location, the temporal artery."

"What does that mean?"

"I'm concerned that you have a disease called Giant Cell Arteritis. It's a rare disease, but there is severe inflammation of the arteries of the head and brain."

"Are you sure about this?" Tommy asked.

"It sounds like a pretty serious diagnosis, just on the basis of a few questions and a physical exam," Agatha added, doubtfully.

I nodded.

"We need to do some blood tests and also a biopsy of the tender artery in your right temple to really nail the diagnosis," I said.

"How are we going to do those things? Can we do them in Hotspur?"

"No, we probably need to send you to Abilene or Dallas."

"Is this a serious condition?"

"Yes. The inflammation in the arteries can make them swell up so much that they cut off circulation. I'm particularly concerned about the loss of vision."

"It was just temporary. I'm back to normal now," Agatha said.

"I know. But it can come back and next time you might not be so lucky. This disease can cause sudden permanent blindness and strokes."

Tommy and Agatha gaped.

"Well, we can go wherever you want," Tommy said. "Whenever you want. We can leave first thing tomorrow morning."

"No, it's not that simple. This is actually a medical emergency. Agatha could go blind with this disease and it could strike again in the next few hours. She needs to start the treatment *right now.*"

"But we haven't done the tests to check for it!"

"Yes, but it's Saturday night and we're in Hotspur. We're miles from a big hospital and it could be days before we can make a definitive diagnosis!"

"So what do we do?"

"We need to start steroids right away. I'm going to call Elvis at Owl Drugs to bring you some prednisone tonight."

"Tonight? Are you sure? Are we just making this into a big deal?" Agatha protested.

"Sandy, this is a big deal. Should we do the tests first?" Tommy asked.

I paused. I remembered Karl's advice: *once you make a diagnosis, be utterly confident. Own it! The patient needs to believe you.*

"I'm sure. Absolutely sure! Agatha has giant cell arteritis. She needs prednisone and she needs it tonight. I'm calling the pharmacy right now and she needs to start prednisone immediately."

Tommy looked less doubtful.

"There is a real danger of her going blind in the next few hours!" I repeated, grimly.

Agatha jumped up. Tommy followed.

"I believe you, Sandy. Tommy and I are headed home and I will start the prednisone tonight. I believe you. Please call it in. Elvis goes to our church and he's a good friend. I know he'll deliver it tonight."

I was relieved. I looked at Maya and remained silent.

"Thank you, Doctor," Tommy said. "We've ended meals with chocolates and wine and desserts, but never before with a prescription for steroids! I'm so glad I told you about Agatha's headache before we left!"

"God moves in strange and wondrous ways, His miracles to perform," I repeated. Tommy chuckled.

We shook hands and hugged. The Templars stepped out and walked home briskly.

* * *

The girls bathed quickly and got back into their pajamas. I turned the lights out, and Maya and I sat silently in the corridor outside the girls' room. We listened to the clicking of the fan, the hum of the air conditioner and the churning of the dishwasher. In-between those sounds, we monitored the slow, soft breathing of the children. Drafts of cool air whistled and blended the fragrance of soap and shampoo with the faint smell of rice. I thought about the path we had taken together, from Delhi to London to Houston, and now in Hotspur. Maya, Priya, Anjali and I had come with misgivings, but three years later, we had a home and friends we loved. We didn't want to leave.

"I hope you're right about that diagnosis," Maya whispered .

"I'm pretty sure I'm right."

"Have you seen it before?"

"A couple of times in London."

"Just a *couple* of times?"

"Yes. It's rare."

"Then how did you sound so confident about the diagnosis?" Maya wondered.

"I was pretty sure but I wanted to sound completely confident to reassure Agatha and Tommy."

We heard some rustling and stopped talking for a few minutes.

"What if it's the wrong diagnosis?" Maya hissed.

"I am pretty sure I'm right. And if I'm right then I've saved her from going blind or having a stroke."

"And if you're wrong?"

"Then I've given her a round of steroids for no good reason. But steroids are not that harmful. We can run the tests next week and if I'm wrong, we can stop the steroids. No major long-term problems."

Maya looked at me for a minute then changed the subject.

"The job offer they made you, what a sweet deal! That is so nice of them, to let you take their equipment to other little towns," Maya enthused.

"It really is. Most hospitals would never do that," I agreed.

"I think they really like you here."

"I think so, too."

"Maybe we should stay here awhile. I mean, stay in Hotspur. Maybe try it out," Maya said.

"Try it out? You mean, do GI from town to town with a van full of scopes and medical gear? Do clinics and procedures in a bunch of little towns?"

"It's contrarian, but it could work."

"Yes. I could give it a shot."

"You always like to be contrarian. This would be contrarian," Maya pointed out.

"It looks a little weird. I mean, it looks like a traveling salesman, you know, driving from place to place, lugging your own stuff around, bouncing around in a van like a circus act."

Maya thought for a moment.

"So what if it's not, like, traditional. Why not try it out at least?"

"I might look pretty foolish and desperate. I might look like a big failure, you know. Couldn't get a job in a big city, so went lurching around the countryside in a big beat-up old wagon. I'm going to look stupid."

"No, you're not. What if it succeeds? What if the small towns really like you and you just go there for a week or so, bring your scopes, and the little hospitals get paid the facility fee and the Hotspur hospital makes a nice packet by sharing their equipment. Everyone's happy. "

"I don't know."

"It could succeed. Look at the opportunity they're giving you. They're risking their equipment and nurses for you. Not many people would do that."

"True. But it's still a gamble."

"Coming to America was a gamble. Coming to Hotspur was a gamble."

"Hotspur had a defined job and a clear benefit. This new idea is a long shot, doing something nobody's done before."

"You miss a hundred percent of the shots you don't take, remember?"

I smiled.

"I quote Yogi Berra so much, you're quoting him back to me."

"You should listen to what you say. Sometimes you actually make sense."

"Let's think about it," I said.

* * *

Maya and I crept back to our bedroom and lay there quietly.

"I liked London. I liked walking in Hampstead Heath and Kew Gardens."

"I did enjoy that. We were lucky to live in Hampstead. I really thought we would settle down in London or maybe return to Delhi."

"So did I."

"From Hampstead Heath to Hotspur, Texas. Did you ever dream we would end up here?" I asked.

"Never," Maya said.

"Talking to the Templars, I realize just how lucky I've been. I keep worrying about patients and complications and the hospitals, but I forget that I have the three of you."

Maya shifted.

"It's not always been easy. I know you care for us. But sometimes it feels like all you want to do is medicine," Maya said.

"I get a high when things go well in my practice. It's a strange attraction."

"I want you to remember that you're a dad and a husband and not just The Specialist."

"I'll never forget that."

"So I went to the local jeweler in town, Earle Smith's. I had them make you a new wedding band."

"That's so nice! Thank you."

"Several people in town pointed out that you don't wear one," Maya said. "It really bothers me."

"I kept taking it off to wash my hands and I lost it, in London, and never replaced it."

"I know. But I think you need to try again and make a bigger effort this time. Remember, you have Priya and Anjali and me."

"Is the band here in the bedroom? I want to wear it right now," I said, getting up.

"Yes. I got a tiny inscription on the band, too, you can barely read it," Maya whispered. "I thought you'd like it personalized."

"What is it? What does it say?" I asked.

Maya smiled.

"Love me ever, leave me never," she said.

I grasped her hands and sat down again in the dark and couldn't think of anything more to say. I looked back at the three years we had spent in Hotspur and realized that they had been a blessing. I thought of the day we moved in. I thought of the days Maya had taken the girls to the neighbors and our days biking and picnicking and visiting friends and Maya dancing with me in the parking lot outside the Cattlewomen's Ball, and of the nights I told the girls stories till they fell asleep. I realized how we had all matured in three years. I wanted time to stop right there. I wanted to go back and live those memories again and again and make them last forever.

I stayed awake for some time after Maya slept. My mind wandered.

I thought about the evening, and how Maya and the girls had been so happy and relaxed. Three years ago, just before we were supposed to move to Buffalo, New York, I made a phone call and lost the job. I didn't want to jeopardize our paradise again.

I thought about my diagnosis for Agatha. It was a strange twist of fate that Tommy had mentioned her headaches in passing, and it had such serious implications. I had read extensively about this disease, temporal arteritis, and felt confident about the diagnosis. I was reassured that the treatment was with prednisone, which could cause bothersome side effects, but was not toxic or dangerous. If my diagnosis was wrong, it would not cause her any serious harm. If my diagnosis was correct, it would save her sight and prevent a stroke.

I thought about the hospital board allowing me to take the endoscopes and all the associated equipment with me to perform procedures in other small towns. I knew how many thousands of dollars had been invested in new equipment! I felt humbled and grateful. I thought of Dr. Naunton Morgan and how pleased he would be if I started doing procedures in Abilene. Of course, Dr. Wegener would be furious. And I was okay with that.

I thought of many others I had met in Hotspur. Mark and Amanda Hastings had liked me inspite of my views on evolution, and Sparky and Cactus Leftwich, who had pneumonia and insisted on smoking in the hospital, and the Rutherfords, who had ultimately supported my application for green cards. I remembered Bill Hennessy, who took me in his truck to take care of his friend, Herschel Dunn, when he refused to come to the hospital. I was grateful for Simon Godwyn and Ben Grimes and Penny Merriwether and Hawkeye. The awesome Dell Clawsom had become a good friend and had taken me flying. They had all helped me gain confidence in myself.

I had many teachers and professors, but my latest was Karl Becker. He was blessed with knowledge and ability, and his skills were burnished with confidence. He was also blunt and prickly and had to be handled with respect and caution. But he had taught me so much. I saw him in my mind, sauntering along the rocky edge of Hord's Creek Lake, after that stunning performance on his jet ski.

I thought about Maya and Priya and Anjali, and how we had come to Hotspur three years ago in a nearly empty Mayflower truck. We had survived the first year, managed to get our green cards the second year, and come into our own the third year. We were fortunate. I knew several colleagues who were still stuck in the immigration process.

I was more confident in myself as a doctor and I was grateful to the people of Hotspur for giving me a chance and encouraging me. I thought of the Washingtons, who still followed up with me and never mentioned the perforation. I thought of our neighbors, especially Priya's friend, Aubrey, who had been hit by a falling TV and I had air-flighted to Dallas.

I was welcome here. I was not welcome in Abilene, at least, not right now. Why not try to practice as a specialist in the small towns of West Texas? I could remain based in Hotspur, so we wouldn't have to uproot ourselves again. We could drive to Abilene and Dallas and Austin whenever we wished.

No one had done anything like this before, but it could work. I would be able to stay in rural Texas, with its wide-open spaces, its mesquites, pecans, and oaks, and pale green plains studded with limestone and yucca and cacti and cattle, and work with people who wanted me to stay. I had always imagined myself in a large teaching hospital in London or Houston, but three years in Hotspur had changed my outlook completely.

I had never imagined living in the heart of Texas, yet here we were, settled and comfortable. Maybe I was never destined to be an academician or a scientist, just a father, husband, and doctor.

I remembered part of Tommy's prayer. *Thank You for bringing us to this part of Paradise.*

I looked out the bay window and gazed at the fence and the trees gilded with moonlight and the stars glittering in the cosmos. These very constellations had illuminated my path since I was born and seemed to be guiding me through voyages I had never imagined. There they would remain, to guide others long after me. I prayed and fell asleep, reassured, knowing that there was a greater power watching over all of us.

The End.